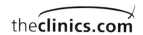

NURSING CLINICS
OF NORTH AMERICA

Alzheimer's Disease

GUEST EDITOR
Ivo L. Abraham, PhD, RN, CS, FAAN

March 2006 • Volume 41 • Number 1

SAUNDERS

An Imprint of Elsevier, Inc.
PHILADELPHIA   LONDON   TORONTO   MONTREAL   SYDNEY   TOKYO

W.B. SAUNDERS COMPANY
A Division of Elsevier Inc.

1600 John F. Kennedy Blvd., Suite 1800, Philadelphia, PA 19103-2899

http://www.theclinics.com

NURSING CLINICS OF NORTH AMERICA
March 2006
Editor: Maria Lorusso

Volume 41, Number 1
ISSN 0029-6465
ISBN 1-4160-3534-6

The ideas and opinions expressed in *Nursing Clinics of North America* do not necessarily reflect those of the Publisher. The Publisher does not assume any responsibility for any injury and/or damage to persons or property arising out of or related to any use of the material contained in this periodical. The reader is advised to check the appropriate medical literature and the product information currently provided by the manufacturer of each drug to be administered to verify the dosage, the method and duration of administration, or contraindications. It is the responsibility of the treating physician or other health care professional, relying on independent experience and knowledge of the patient, to determine drug dosages and the best treatment for the patient. Mention of any product in this issue should not be construed as endorsement by the contributors, editors, or the Publisher of the product or manufacturers' claims.

Nursing Clinics of North America (ISSN 0029-6465) is published quarterly by W.B. Saunders, 360 Park Avenue South, New York, NY 10010-1710. Months of publication are March, June, September, and December. Business and Editorial Offices: 1600 John F. Kennedy Blvd., Suite 1800, Philadelphia, PA 19103-2899. Accounting and Circulation Offices: 6277 Sea Harbor Drive, Orlando, FL 32887-4800. Periodicals postage paid at New York, NY and additional mailing offices. Subscription price per year is, $105.00 (US individuals), $200.00 (US institutions), $170.00 (international individuals), $240.00 (international institutions), $145.00 (Canadian individuals), $240.00 (Canadian institutions), $55.00 (US students), and $85.00 (international students). To receive student/resident rate, orders must be accompanied by name of affiliated institution, date of term, and the signature of program/residency coordinator on institution letterhead. Orders will be billed at individual rate until proof of status is received. Foreign air speed delivery is included in all *Clinics* subscription prices. All prices are subject to change without notice. **POSTMASTER:** Send address changes to *Nursing Clinics of North America*, Elsevier Periodicals Customer Service, 6277 Sea Harbor Drive, Orlando, FL 32887-4800. **Customer Service: 1-800-654-2452 (US). From outside of the US, call 1-407-345-4000.**

Nursing Clinics of North America is covered in *EMBASE/Excerpta Medica, Index Medicus, Social Sciences Citation Index, Current Contents, ASCA, Cumulative Index to Nursing, R.Ndex Top 100,* and *Allied Health Literature and International Nursing Index (INI).*

Printed in the United States of America.

NURSING CLINICS
OF NORTH AMERICA

Alzheimer's Disease

GUEST EDITOR

IVO L. ABRAHAM, PhD, RN, CS, FAAN, Principal, Matrix45, Earlysville, Virginia and Heverlee, Belgium; Adjunct Professor, Center for Health Outcomes and Policy Research, School of Nursing & Leonard Davis Institute of Health Economics, Wharton School of Business, University of Pennsylvania, Philadelphia, Pennsylvania; Adjunct Clinical Professor, College of Nursing, University of Arizona, Tucson, Arizona; Adjunct Clinical Professor, School of Nursing, New York University, New York, New York; Adjunct Professor, School of Nursing, University of Virginia, Charlottesville, Virginia

CONTRIBUTORS

IVO L. ABRAHAM, PhD, RN, CS, FAAN, Principal, Matrix45, Earlysville, Virginia and Heverlee, Belgium; Adjunct Professor, Center for Health Outcomes and Policy Research, School of Nursing & Leonard Davis Institute of Health Economics, Wharton School of Business, University of Pennsylvania, Philadelphia, Pennsylvania; Adjunct Clinical Professor, College of Nursing, University of Arizona, Tucson, Arizona; Adjunct Clinical Professor, School of Nursing, New York University, New York, New York; Adjunct Professor, School of Nursing, University of Virginia, Charlottesville, Virginia

TOM BRAES, MSN, RN, Research Fellow, Centre for Health Services and Nursing Research, Katholieke Universiteit Leuven; Clinical Nurse Specialist, Department of Geriatrics, University Hospitals of Leuven, Leuven, Belgium

KATHLEEN C. BUCKWALTER, PhD, RN, Professor, University of Iowa College of Nursing, Iowa City, Iowa

VALERIE T. COTTER, MSN, CRNP, FAANP, Program Director, Adult Health and Gerontology Nurse Practitioner Programs, School of Nursing, University of Pennsylvania, Philadelphia, Pennsylvania

ANNE DEBLANDER, MD, Medical Manager, Novartis Pharma Belgium, Vilvoorde, Belgium

DONNA M. FICK, PhD, APRN-BC, Associate Professor, School of Nursing, College of Health and Human Development, The Pennsylvania State University; School of Medicine, Department of Psychiatry, The Pennsylvania State University, University Park, Pennsylvania

MARQUIS D. FOREMAN, PhD, RN, FAAN, Professor and Associate Dean for Nursing Science Studies, College of Nursing, University of Illinois at Chicago, Chicago, Illinois

TERRY FULMER, PhD, RN, FAAN, The Erline Perkins McGriff Professor and Head, Division of Nursing, New York University, New York, New York

LINDA GERDNER, PhD, RN, Assistant Professor, University of Minnesota School of Nursing, Minneapolis, Minnesota

GERI RICHARDS HALL, PhD, ARNP, CNS, FAAN, Clinical Professor and Advanced Practice Nurse, University of Iowa College of Nursing and Medicine, Iowa City, Iowa

KAREN M. MACDONALD, PhD, RN, Principal, Matrix 45, Earlysville, Virginia and Heverlee, Belgium

KOEN MILISEN, PhD, RN, Assistant Professor, Centre for Health Services and Nursing Research, Katholieke Universiteit Leuven; Clinical Nurse Specialist, Department of Geriatrics, University Hospitals of Leuven, Leuven, Belgium

DEBORAH M. NADZAM, PhD, RN, FAAN, Director, Institute for Healthcare Quality, The Cleveland Clinic Health System; Adjunct Professor, Frances Payne Bolton School of Nursing, Case Western Reserve University, Cleveland, Ohio

LISA L. ONEGA, PhD, RN, FNP, CNS, GNP, Associate Professor of Gerontological Nursing, Radford University, Radford, Virginia

GREGORY J. PAVEZA, MSW, PhD, Director, Division of Arts and Sciences, University of South Florida, Lakeland, Florida

MARIANNE SMITH, PhD(c), ARNP, CS, John A. Hartford Scholar, Predoctoral Fellow, University of Iowa College of Nursing, Iowa City, Iowa

STEFAAN VANCAYZEELE, MD, Chief Medical Officer, Novartis Pharma Belgium, Vilvoorde, Belgium

CARLA VANDEWEERD, PhD, Associate Director, The James and Jennifer Harrell Center, Department of Community and Family Health, College of Public Health, University of South Florida, Tampa, Florida

NURSING CLINICS
OF NORTH AMERICA

ELSEVIER
SAUNDERS

Alzheimer's Disease

CONTENTS

VOLUME 41 • NUMBER 1 • MARCH 2006

Preface
Ivo L. Abraham

xi

**Cognitive Assessment and Differentiating the 3 Ds
(Dementia, Depression, Delirium)**
Koen Milisen, Tom Braes, Donna M. Fick, and
Marquis D. Foreman

1

Differentiation between a diminished or altered cognitive functioning as
a consequence of aging and one resulting from serious health problems
is critical in the elderly. An unrecognized cognitive disorder or the worsening of the impairment may hamper the effectiveness and appropriateness of care and treatment; therefore, standardized assessment
procedures and systematic monitoring of cognition and behavior are
important aspects of the nursing care of older adults. In this article, current notions for accurate and comprehensive cognitive assessment in
older persons are delineated. Further, an overview of epidemiological
screening and diagnostic dilemmas of dementia, depression, and delirium
are provided.

**Assessment of Psychoemotional and Behavioral
Status in Patients with Dementia**
Lisa L. Onega

23

Depression and behavioral symptoms occur in many older adults with
dementia and result in serious consequences, including nursing home
admissions, decreased functional ability, mortality, and increased health
care costs. Assessment of depression in this population is challenging
and is facilitated by using interviewer-rated instruments as an adjunct
to clinical judgment. Clinicians should select a perspective that enables
them to view behavioral symptoms associated with dementia in a therapeutic manner. Care for depression and behavioral symptoms should
be individualized to match presenting symptoms. Issues related to psychoemotional and behavioral assessment are: (1) implementation of
effective psychogeriatric models of care and (2) incorporating evidenced-
based knowledge into practice settings.

**Abuse and Neglect in Older Adults with
Alzheimer's Disease**
Carla VandeWeerd, Gregory J. Paveza, and Terry Fulmer

43

Elder mistreatment is a serious issue that effects the lives of thousands
of older adults and results in emotional difficulties, such as depression,

feelings of inadequacy, self-loathing, and lowered self-esteem. It has been shown to result in family distress, impaired life functioning, and difficulties with cognition and has been linked to health problems, such as immunologic dysfunction, and increased mortality. As the population ages, and with it the numbers of persons afflicted by diseases such as Alzheimer's, understanding and recognizing elder mistreatment becomes an important factor in maintaining quality of life for older adults.

Application of the Progressively Lowered Stress Threshold Model Across the Continuum of Care   57
Marianne Smith, Geri Richards Hall, Linda Gerdner, and Kathleen C. Buckwalter

Over the last two decades, increasing attention has been paid to the nature of behavioral symptoms in dementia. Early notions that all behaviors were an inevitable component of cognitive impairment have all but disappeared in the face of evidence that diverse personal, social, and environmental factors regularly act as antecedents to behavioral and psychologic symptoms of dementia (BPSD). The quality of care provided to persons with dementia has been advanced through nursing care conceptual models that explain antecedents to BPSD and, in turn, offer specific interventions to promote comfort and optimal function.

Alzheimer's Disease: Issues and Challenges in Primary Care   83
Valerie T. Cotter

The challenge in primary care practice is identifying persons with symptoms of Alzheimer's Disease (AD) who often have limited capacity to recognize their own symptoms and attribute cognitive decline to chronic illness or aging. Brief office visit communications without an informant, such as a spouse or adult child rarely uncover mild stage AD. Clinicians in primary care fail to screen older adults for AD on a routine basis because of insufficient time, inadequate reimbursement for services, and uncertainty about the value of an early diagnosis. Although current pharmacologic and behavioral interventions and patient education do not prevent eventual disease progression, they arguably lead to improvements in understanding, self-efficacy, and quality of life for the patient and family.

Measuring the Quality of Nursing Care to Alzheimer's Patients   95
Ivo L. Abraham, Karen M. MacDonald, and Deborah M. Nadzam

Facilities that provide care to Alzheimer's disease patients are under unrelenting pressure to document the quality of nursing care they provide to various stakeholders. Unfortunately, little consensus exists nor is guidance given as to how to measure the quality of nursing care. Regulations and standards exist but are seldom translated into systematic outcome measures that assist nurses and facilities to measure, report, and manage the quality of care they provide to residents in general and Alzheimer's patients in particular. This article offers practical advice on conceptualizing quality of nursing care to Alzheimer's patients and the selection of outcome measures to collect, analyze, use, and report quality of nursing care data.

Longitudinal Observational Studies to Study the Efficacy-Effectiveness Gap in Drug Therapy: Application to Mild and Moderate Dementia 105
Karen M. MacDonald, Stefaan Vancayzeele, Anne Deblander, and Ivo L. Abraham

If well-designed, longitudinal observational studies (LOSs) can provide insights to the linkages between real-world outcomes and their multilevel determinants. In this article, some of the scientific and methodologic issues related to LOSs in pharmacotherapeutic evaluations are discussed. A case of such a study in the treatment of mild to moderate dementia is provided—a case in which a pharmaceutic sponsor addressing a medical question (long-term effectiveness) realized that caring for patients who have Alzheimer's disease involves the clinical community of caregivers, physicians, families, nurses, psychologists, and pharmacists, among others, and partnered with nurse researchers to design their inquiry. The authors conclude by presenting an argument for nurses to take the lead in effectiveness research.

Dementia and Alzheimer's Disease: A Practical Orientation 119
Ivo L. Abraham

This article presents a functional, brief, and, above all, practical orientation to Alzheimer's disease. This disease, with its many unanswered questions (and occasional unquestioned answers), is in first instance a disease to be cared for. The burden of this caring initially falls on caregivers and families; however, once Alzheimer's patients enter the formal health care system, nurses will be at the forefront of care. The foundation to good care is a solid but also applied understanding of the disease, how it manifests itself, and how it is experienced by patients, caregivers, and families.

Erratum 129

Index 131

NURSING CLINICS
OF NORTH AMERICA

FORTHCOMING ISSUES

June 2006

Perioperative Nursing
Gratia Nagle, RN, BA, CNOR, CRNFA, *Guest Editor*

September 2006

HIV/AIDS Update
Yvonne Wesley, PhD, RN, *Guest Editor*

December 2006

Diabetes
Gail D'Eramo Melkus, EdD, C-ANP, CDE, FAAN, *Guest Editor*

RECENT ISSUES

December 2005

School-Based Health Centers and Nurse-Managed Health Centers
Judith Scully, PhD, RN, CCNS, Diana Hackbarth, PhD, RN, FAAN, and
Barbara Rideout, MSN, APRN, BC, *Guest Editors*

September 2005

Disaster Management and Response
Judith Stoner Halpern, MS, NP, APRN, BC and
Mary W. Chaffee, ScD (hon), MS, RN, CNAA, FAAN,
Guest Editors

June 2005

Wound Care
Barbara Pieper, PhD, RN, CS, CWOCN, FAAN, *Guest Editor*

Nurs Clin N Am 41 (2006) xi–xiii

NURSING CLINICS
OF NORTH AMERICA

PREFACE

Alzheimer's Disease

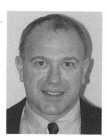

Ivo L. Abraham, PhD, RN, CS, FAAN

Guest Editor

Alzheimer's disease has become a familiar if not feared concept within the general public and among health care professionals. We now know a lot more about it; we realize how devastating the disease can be; and we recognize how taxing it can be on caregivers, families, and health care providers. As research and scholarship in nursing as well as the health and social sciences has grown in volume, breadth, and depth, our understanding of disease, patients and caregivers, and interventions has gained. Where once we may have studied some clinical Alzheimer's issue from a broad perspective, increasing specialization can now be detected. In the process, the potential knowledge base has grown by leaps and bounds—only to present researchers and clinicians with the challenge of synthesis and integration.

This present issue of the *Nursing Clinics of North America* is the third on Alzheimer's disease that I have had the pleasure of editing. In 1988, Kitty Buckwalter at the University of Iowa, and Marcia Neundorfer and I at Case Western Reserve University, attempted to lay a foundation for nursing as the profession found itself increasingly thrust to the forefront of care to patients and caregivers. We chose what, in retrospect, looks like a classical approach: definition of Alzheimer's disease; how to care for patients at home, in the community, and in long-term care facilities; effect on caregivers and families; the person–environment interaction; emerging nursing interventions; and the link to psychiatry. The focus was on synthesis, the goal to further the understanding of clinicians.

In 1994, a second issue of the *Nursing Clinics of North America* was dedicated to Alzheimer's disease. A key realization was the growth in research and clinical

0029-6465/06/$ – see front matter
doi:10.1016/j.cnur.2005.11.001

scholarship in a relatively short time. A focus on synthesis remained; we wanted to bring together new insights, developments, and trends in function of supporting clinical nursing practice. There was also an implicit aim of setting direction and stimulating interdisciplinary collaboration. Thus, the 1994 issue addressed new insights in the disease and its epidemiology; focused on comprehensive assessment; behavioral management, both indirectly and directly; the design of care environments; and interventions for and with caregivers.

Now it is 2006, 18 years after the initial issue and 12 years after the second. What can we contribute to clinical nursing at this time? As this issue was being planned in late 2004, a continued focus on synthesis seemed important but not essential; in fact, there are many sources available for multiple target audiences. Trying to provide a comprehensive synthesis seemed less urgent, let alone practical within the space of a typical *Nursing Clinics* issue. Furthermore, with the burgeoning literature and the explosion of electronic sources, much knowledge and evidence is readily accessible. Perhaps too much knowledge and evidence, thus creating the need for filtration, focusing, and next-stage focusing–the aims eventually embedded in this third issue.

The need for filtration is emphasized in the first article, where I try to bring to the forefront the "bare" issues of dementia and Alzheimer's disease as they apply to clinical nursing practice. A rather exhaustive search of the literature and the internet yielded a divergent mixture of resources – from the theoretical to the practical, the superficial to the deep, the scientific to the applied. At the risk of producing a seemingly simplistic paper, the attempt was to focus functionally and practically on the "signs and symptoms" as they might affect the dynamics of nursing care to patients and families.

It also seemed time for direction in differentiated assessment. Milisen and colleagues translate the evidence base on the "three D's" (Delirium, Dementia, Depression) into structured guidance for differentiated assessment of cognitive impairment. In her article, Onega focuses on assessment in the psychoemotional sphere, drawing on both quantitative and qualitative research. A perhaps novel addition is the article by Vandeweerd and colleagues on the assessment of elder mistreatment–still an underrecognized problem in the care of patients who have cognitive impairment.

The Progressively Lowered Stress Threshold (PLST) model has been a guiding principle for the past 20 years in the care of patients who have Alzheimer's disease and dementia. Under the lead of Smith, the Iowa group that developed the model and built much of the evidence base for it contributes an article that underscores the integration of the PLST in daily clinical practice. It has been rewarding personally to see the PLST progress from concept to hypothesis to evidence and, eventually, to implicit standard of care.

With the growth in advanced nursing practice, it seemed important to assist practitioners in the detection and management of Alzheimer's in primary care. Cotter relies upon her experience and expertise, clinical and academic, to provide direction to a group of clinicians often ill-prepared to face the challenges of caring for Alzheimer's patients and their families.

Another new area of attention is the need for evaluating the care provided by nurses and developing frameworks for studying the determinants and outcomes of care. Abraham and colleagues provide practical advice on how to evaluate the quality of nursing care to patients who have Alzheimer's disease using outcome measures as indicators of performance. MacDonald and colleagues review issues in studying the effectiveness of interventions by linking outcomes to determinants at different levels of care.

One can only hope that this present issue of the *Nursing Clinics of North America* will indeed contribute to better nursing care for Alzheimer's patients and their families. We began the preface to the 1988 issue with the following quote from Arnold Toynbee: "A society's quality and durability can best be measured by the respect and care given its elderly citizens." Much may have changed in our knowledge base on the care of Alzheimer's disease over the past 20 years or so—the responsibility hasn't.

Ivo L. Abraham, PhD, RN, CS, FAAN
Matrix45
620 Frays Ridge Road
Earlysville, VA 22936, USA

E-mail address: iabraham@matrix45.com

Nurs Clin N Am 41 (2006) 1–22

NURSING CLINICS
OF NORTH AMERICA

Cognitive Assessment and Differentiating the 3 Ds (Dementia, Depression, Delirium)

Koen Milisen, PhD, RN[a,b,*], Tom Braes, MSN, RN[a,b],
Donna M. Fick, PhD, APRN-BC[c,d],
Marquis D. Foreman, PhD, RN, FAAN[e]

[a]Centre for Health Services and Nursing Research, Katholieke Universiteit Leuven,
Kapucijnenvoer 35/4, 3000 Leuven, Belgium
[b]Department of Geriatrics, University Hospitals of Leuven, Leuven, Belgium
[c]College of Health and Human Development, School of Nursing, The Pennsylvania
State University, University Park, PA, USA
[d]School of Medicine, Department of Psychiatry, The Pennsylvania State University,
University Park, PA, USA
[e]College of Nursing, University of Illinois at Chicago, Chicago, IL, USA

Cognitive functioning, the processes of perceiving, registering, storing and using information change with aging [1–4]. The loss of recent memory, a delayed response time, and a diminished ability to learn complex information are examples of physiologic, rather than pathologic, changes that occur with ageing [2,4]. Cognitive conditions like dementia, delirium, and depression represent serious pathologic impairments requiring detailed assessment and specific treatments. Nevertheless, diminished or altered cognitive functioning is perceived by health care professionals often routinely as a normal or logical consequence of ageing. This negative ageist stereotype results in a myriad of unconstructive outcomes. An unrecognized cognitive disorder or the worsening of impairment may hamper the effectiveness of necessary treatment or interventions, possibly postponing discharge in the case of hospitalization. A lack of attention for the evaluation and documentation of a patient's cognitive status may compromise the possible reversibility of some cognitive disorders (eg, some aspects of delirium, secondary types of dementia). Additionally, when inaccurately assessed, the individual's cognitive decline may be misdiagnosed, resulting in the implementation of incorrect therapeutic intervention [2]. Furthermore, because the individual's abilities (cognitive and physical) were never thoroughly mapped, the patient is deprived of individualized care or revalidation necessary to maximize his remaining abilities.

*Corresponding author. E-mail address: koen.milisen@med.kuleuven.be (K. Milisen).

0029-6465/06/$ – see front matter
doi:10.1016/j.cnur.2005.09.001

Besides the above-mentioned clinical examples and the obvious economic repercussions (eg, increased length of stay, increased use of resources), it is important to realize that health care professionals, in particular nurses, also benefit from integrating cognitive assessment in their daily practice. Although evaluating a patient's cognitive status is often seen as being time consuming, the "net time-investment" of doing so outweighs the perceived disadvantages. The patient's behavior can then be comprehended; the results of the assessment make it possible to communicate in a uniform way with colleagues and physicians (as the results of the assessment offer a standardized "language"); the evolution of the patient's cognitive abilities can be measured and compared; and, last, but equally important, for the older person's relatives the behavior of the patient can be explained or clarified [5]. Finally, to emphasize the importance of cognitive assessment, it is essential to bear in mind that especially in older persons (acute) cognitive decline may be the first signal that something's wrong (eg, urinary incontinence, dehydration, functional decline) an indicator that rigorous assessment is needed.

The purpose of this article is to delineate current notions regarding accurate and comprehensive cognitive assessment in older persons. More specifically, the authors address different purposes of cognitive assessment, caveats to consider when selecting an assessment instrument and instructions on how to perform and interpret results of the assessment. Further, the authors summarize epidemiology, clinical features, risk factors, areas of assessment, and examples of instruments for three of the most significant cognitive disorders occurring in older people: dementia, depression, and delirium.

COGNITIVE ASSESSMENT
Defining the Purpose of Assessment
The term "cognitive assessment" has to be seen as a generic or an "umbrella term," representing four different approaches ranging from broad to detailed and each with its specific purpose: screening, diagnosis, monitoring, or a combination of one of these purposes [1,6]. As a first step, it is of major importance to define the required focus. Screening, for a start, is conducted simply to determine whether or not a cognitive impairment is present, so relative imprecise methods are acceptable. Screening tests tend to be brief, containing only essential items and requiring further in-depth evaluation to confirm the exact problem and its etiology. Diagnostic methods provide more precise and detailed information about the patient's cognitive status. The methods can be used to identify the precise nature and cause of the cognitive impairment and to determine the remaining cognitive abilities of the individual [1,6]. Monitoring, at last, intends to determine the individual's cognitive functioning over time—when evaluating the response to treatment, for instance [1].

Selecting the Instrument
When selecting an instrument, factors, in addition to the purpose of the assessment, should be considered: the time required for administration (for patients

and raters); the level of rater expertise and training required to reliably administer an instrument and interpret results; the subpopulation the instrument is designed for; and the psychometric properties of the test [7].

Instruments come in all shapes and sizes; ranging from brief, one-dimensional instruments assessing only a single cognitive process to the full-scale batteries providing an overall indication of the patient's cognitive status [1]. Each type has its advantages and disadvantages. Large, multidimensional instruments often require a skilled examiner, place intense demands on the patient, and may be less sensitive to some aspects of cognition. The brief instruments, although usable at the bedside and less demanding on the examiner and examinee, may overlook a crucial deficit in one of the cognitive processes simply by focusing solely on one specific component (eg, attention) [1].

Another aspect that has to be verified is the (sub) population the instrument initially was designed for, as the instrument may need to be modified to accommodate certain characteristics of the (sub) population, such as educational level, race, and presence of vision and hearing impairments or underlying diseases. Finally, depending on the purpose of the assessment, demands concerning the psychometric properties (eg, sensitivity and specificity) of the test vary. As a rule of thumb, for screening purposes—being the most relevant for bedside nurses—an instrument is valid if it detects most people who have the target disorder (high sensitivity) and excludes most patients who do not have the disorder (high specificity) and if a positive test usually indicates that the disorder is present (high positive predictive value) [8]. By briefly searching the available literature, the necessary information is available to determine if the selected instrument has satisfactory psychometric properties. Given these additional aspects that have to be considered, selecting the most appropriate instrument is about making a well-considered choice.

Conducting the Assessment

In conducting the assessment, the following should be considered: the physical environment, the interpersonal environment, and some points of interest regarding the preferred moment of assessing [1]. Concerning the physical environment, the privacy for the examiner and the examinee should be guaranteed. The room should be well lit (but not glaring), set at a comfortable ambient temperature, and free from distractions (eg, the assessment should be conducted in the absence of others and other activities) [1,9]. The examinee should be positioned in a comfortable way that maximizes sensory abilities. Regarding the interpersonal environment it is vital to prepare the examinee for the assessment by explaining to the patient what will take place and how long it will take, therefore reducing the examinee's possible anxiety and creating an emotionally nonthreatening environment and a safe patient-professional relationship [1,9]. Furthermore, during the assessment the examiner should respect the pace or rate of response set by the patient, paying attention to possible signs of fatigue (eg, slurring of speech, restlessness). Dividing the assessment in different sections/sessions or temporally terminating the assessment should be considered in case of fatigue. When selecting the most suitable moment for assessing the patient's cognitive status, the following times of the day should generally be avoided: immediately on awakening from sleep (wait at least 30 minutes), immediately before and after meals, immediately before and after medical diagnostic or therapeutic procedures, and those moments when the patient experiences pain or discomfort. Following these guidelines, the assessment will be valid and reliable, reflecting the individual's cognitive abilities without interference by any extraneous factors.

Besides the above-mentioned steps, the success of the (cognitive) assessment greatly depends on the examiner's social skills, familiarity with the selected instrument, and capacity to recognize issues that can negatively bias the results. Accurately documenting the results and incorporating them in to daily practice and individualized care plans is essential.

Interpreting the Results of the Assessment

The result and the course of the assessment can be interpreted in a quantitative or a qualitative way. The quantitative approach ("focusing on the figures") implies that the results of the individual's assessment are compared with the representative or normal norm for a specific test, taking into account the known cut-off values. From the quantitative perspective, the results of the assessment also can be used to map the individual's evolution regarding the examinee's cognitive disorder (eg, monitoring cognitive functioning).

The qualitative approach is a case of "reading between the lines," and goes beyond the numeric result. In qualitative perspective, aspects, such as educational level, mood, the choice of words, the overall appearance, health or disease consciousness, attention, and concentration or personal hygiene, also are interpreted during the assessment [1]. Obviously, a "joined" perspective is the most suitable way of interpreting the results.

Although the importance of formally assessing the individual's cognitive status has to be emphasized, it is crucial not to neglect the value of the informal natural way in which nurses gather information about patients (eg, during baths or meals or regular care). Because actual performance is an important assessment finding, this informal way ideally completes the formal assessment, adding different pieces to the overall picture of the patient.

DEMENTIA

Epidemiology

Dementia prevalence ranges from 11% to 28% in persons 65 years of age and older and as high as 50% in persons in their 80s [10]. Alzheimer's disease (AD) is the most common and well known of all the dementias. By 2050, 14 million older persons in the United States are expected to have Alzheimer's dementia [11]. Dementia prevalence in Europe ranges from 5.9% to 9.4% in persons 65 years of age and older, to well over 30% in the over 90 age group [12,13]. Furthermore, AD accounts for 60% to 90% of all cases of dementia. Other forms of dementia to assess include vascular dementia (stepwise deterioration and history of vascular disease), dementia with Lewy bodies (Parkinsonism, hallucinations, sensitivity to neuroleptics), and frontotemporal dementia (earlier onset, loss of insight and inhibition). AD is being recognized increasingly as a major contributor to increased mortality and morbidity in older adults. AD accounted for 21.4 deaths per 100,000 people in the United States in 2003, an increase of 5.9% since 2002 [14], and has increased from number 11 to number 8 as a leading cause of death. Further, dementia is associated with increased morbidity and many associated problems, such as disturbing behaviors, caregiver distress, motor vehicle accidents, and increased health care use [15–17]. Dementia is associated with increased rates of depression and delirium leading to poor prognostic outcomes, though it is unclear whether they are independent risk factors for dementia or a consequence of the dementia. The prevalence rates of delirium and depression superimposed on dementia range from 22% to 89% and from 18% to 35%, respectively [16,18,19]. Further, persons with dementia are at high risk for hospitalization and worsening of their condition. The cost of dementia is substantial. The annual per person costs of AD have been shown to be at least $30,000 depending on whether direct medical costs, informal care, and societal costs are included [20,21]. The Alzheimer's Association has estimated the costs of AD to businesses in the United States exceed $61 billion, including the costs of health care for persons with AD and the cost of caregiving, lost productivity, and absenteeism for United States workers [22]. A review study by Jönsson and Berr [23] found that the cost of dementia in Euros (2004) ranges from 6000 to about 19,000 annually per person costs, including medical and nonmedical costs.

Clinical Features

Dementia is the general term used for a form of cognitive impairment that is chronic, progressive, and occurring over a period of months to years. The primary deficit in dementia is impaired short-term memory that progresses to impaired use of language, impaired ability to function in activities of daily living, and eventually to death. The course of dementia is usually a slow insidious progression over a period of months to years rather than days to weeks. The clinical features of dementia in the early stages may be subtle. Early in the course of the disease individuals may have difficulty with executive functioning tasks, such as balancing their checkbook or carrying out the duties of their job. Impaired short-term memory is often the first sign, but dementia may also include other signs, such as forgetting of appointments, poor personal hygiene, disorganized thoughts, impaired ability to conduct one's job, sexually inappropriate behavior, difficulty shopping, difficulty in driving, spatial deficits, difficulty in new situations or learning new material, and demonstrating poor judgment or socially inappropriate dress or conduct.

The past century has seen considerable progress in the diagnosis of AD, yet the clinical diagnosis is often still one of exclusion. A complete physical examination (with special emphasis on cardiac and nervous systems), and a battery of laboratory and imaging tests are usually done to rule out other conditions.

The focus away from age as criteria for AD and the popular idea of aging and cognitive decline helped health care professionals to move away from terms such as "senility" and "organic brain syndrome" to the construction and embracing of AD as a disease with specific pathologic characteristics and mechanisms. The diagnosis of dementia involves determining whether memory problems represent normal aging, mild cognitive impairment (MCI), delirium, depression, or a true dementia. Though normal aging is believed to result in a decline in mental processing, speed, and difficulty in learning new things, it should not result in changes or impairment in daily functioning, so a comprehensive examination and assessment of physical and mental functioning is needed. The most widely used diagnostic criteria are the National Institute of Neurological and Communicative Disorders and Stroke-Alzheimer's Disease and Related Disorders Association (NINCDS-ADRDA) criteria [24] and the Diagnostic and Statistical Manual of Mental Disorders, Fourth Edition, Text Revision (DSM-IV-TR) criteria [25]. A dementia of the Alzheimer's type is diagnosed according to DSM-IV-TR criteria if memory impairment and one or more of the following are present: disturbed language (aphasia), impaired motor abilities despite intact motor function (apraxia), failure to recognize or identify familiar objects (agnosia), or a disturbance in executive functioning. Additionally, the deficits must result in a decline in functioning and be characterized by a gradual onset with continued decline [25]. These deficits must also not be caused by another underlying progressive central nervous system disorder, systemic conditions known to cause dementia (such as hypothyroidism, human immunodeficiency virus infection, and other conditions), or a substance-induced condition. Also, the symptoms may not occur exclusively during the course of a delirium or be better accounted for by another Axis I disorder, such as depression or schizophrenia [25]. MCI is the newest buzzword in dementia practice and research and is believed to be a precursor to AD. Criteria for MCI was originally developed by Petersen and colleagues [26] and includes (1) memory complaints, (2) normal activities of daily living, (3) normal general cognitive function, (4) abnormal memory for age, and (5) not demented.

The past decade has seen considerable progress in the development of imaging in AD, including the almost routine use of positron emission tomography, single photon emission computed tomography, and functional MRI (fMRI) in research and clinical practice [27]. In the past, imaging in dementia was used as part of the process of exclusion to identify tumors or other problems that might account for the patient presentation. Currently, a rapid increase is occurring in the use of imaging for the prediction of dementia. A recent study by Mosconi and colleagues [28] found that altered hippocampal glucose metabolism is found in mild cognitive impairment and AD and was able to discriminate between normal healthy subjects and MCI. The current trend in the clinical diagnosis of dementia is for earlier and earlier pre-clinical diagnosis criteria so that clinicians can offer access to pharmaceutical products aimed at prevention and treatment of AD. Screening and diagnosing dementia continue to be an important focus of research and practice.

Risk Factors

The strongest known risk factor for AD is age with the greatest incidence of AD occurring in older adults in their late 70s and early 80s. The incidence of AD is about 3% at age 65 years old but increases to over 50% in the 85 and older group and 56% in persons older than 90 years old [29]. As our older population continues to increase the prevalence of AD should also increase. Genes (APOE2, APOE3, APOE4) are also a risk factor but are most strongly connected with early-onset AD. Late-onset AD accounts for more than 90% of all cases of AD, and many cases occur in persons who have no clear genetic predisposition. In addition, even those with the APOE4 genotype do not develop AD always, which suggests the need to focus on the interaction of genetics and environmental factors.

Another emerging area of focus in dementia clinical practice and research is the assessment of lifestyle and environmental factors for dementia, such as exercise, diet, and other cardiovascular risk factors. Recent research has found an association between vascular risk factors and the development of AD. Hypertension, hypercholesterolemia, obesity, and elevated levels of inflammatory markers have also been associated with AD [30,31]. It is still unclear, however, whether modifying those factors will make a difference in the development of AD. Research in dementia and exercise is being conducted currently. Other risk factors include Down syndrome [32], low education, and head trauma.

Cognitive Assessment

The key areas of dementia assessment include: patient and family history of the problem, assessment of judgment and safety, social and psychiatric history, review of medications, physical examination (with a focus on general appearance, speech, neurologic, and cardiovascular examination), general mental status assessment, review of laboratory values, and neuro-imaging to rule out a brain tumor, subdural hematoma, stroke, or other causes of dementia. The most common reasons for a "reversible cause of dementia" are medications, depression, and metabolic problems (thyroid or B12) [27,32,33].

Instruments most commonly used in the diagnosis, screening, and staging of dementia include the Folstein Mini-Mental Status Examination (MMSE) [34], Mini-Cog [35] and the Memory Impairment Screen (MIS) [36,37], the Modified Blessed Dementia Rating Scale (MBDRS) [38], the Clinical Dementia Rating Scale (CDR) [39], and the Global Deterioration Scale (Global DS) [40].

The MIS is a 4-item scale that tests delayed free and cued recall and has been found to correlate with postmortem Alzheimer's pathology [41]. The MBDRS is an 11-item scale that assesses prior cognitive functioning by way of caregiver recall. It has been shown in the Helsinki Aging studies and others to discriminate between demented and nondemented subjects and has been used by delirium and dementia experts to establish premorbid cognitive functioning [38]. The CDR rates dementia on a ratio scale of 0–5 from a caregiver interview with 0 being no or slight memory loss with no impairment in daily functioning and 5 being persons who have dementia, are bedridden, and unable to speak. The Global

DS rates the function on a scale of 1–7 and rates global cognition and functional status, such as walking and continence. All of these tests are screening instruments and should be interpreted in light of the entire clinical picture.

DEPRESSION

Epidemiology

Approximately 6% of older people living at home suffer from a major form of depression and 15% from a mild form of depression. These figures can increase to 45% for older people who have a somatic illness or who are hospitalized. For older people in a nursing home, the figures vary from 6% to 26% for the major form and from 11% to 50% for the minor form. Additionally, up to 70% report feelings of depression to the extent that such feelings create problems in their daily activities [42–45]. Despite these high figures, this complaint often remains undetected and untreated [46,47]. Untreated depression has detrimental consequences for the daily activities of the elderly as the condition interferes with their ability to think, sleep, and eat, as well as with their ability to maintain and keep up social contact. Depression leads to reduced physical activity, deconditioning, and pain and is associated with extended hospital stays and an increased number of readmissions [48,49]. Depression is also a risk factor for noncompliance with medical treatment and can impact negatively on recovery during hospitalization. It can also lead to increased mortality. Suicide is probably the greatest cause of this high level of mortality in the depressed elderly [49]. These serious consequences can be prevented if the disorder is detected quickly, as depression in older people is a psychiatric disorder that is straightforward to treat.

Clinical Features

The symptoms of depression are conventionally divided into three groups: the affective symptoms (eg, depressive state of mind characterized by arrhythmia, asthenia and lack of drive, disinterest in activities enjoyed previously), the cognitive symptoms (eg, slowing down, interference with the ability to think and predominantly negative thoughts) and the somatic symptoms (eg, shortness of breath, poor appetite, constipation, slowing down of the peristaltic movement, fatigue and insomnia). The specific diagnostic value of somatic disorders in older people with depression is low, because they frequently also occur in the nondepressive elderly and in patients who experience somatic illness [50]. It is, therefore, important to pay particular attention to the affective and cognitive symptoms of depression in older people to be able to detect the problem properly [49]. Furthermore, it is important to differentiate between a significant depression and normal short-term reactions (such as grief and distress) occurring, for example, because of a bereavement, a serious financial setback, or a painful illness [45].

The DSM-IV distinguishes between "major depressive disorder," "dysthymia," and "depression not otherwise specified" [25]. In addition to this, three forms of depression occur that often result in misdiagnoses in older patients: somatically "masked" depression, "depressive-pseudodementia," and psychotic depression [51].

A "major depressive disorder" is diagnosed if one single episode or several recurrent "major" depressive episodes occur [25]. In such cases, at least one core symptom (depressed mood or loss of interest or pleasure) persists throughout the greater part of the day and over a period of at least two weeks. The depressive state of mind is characterized predominantly by a sad, hopeless, demoralized, or even irritable feeling. This feeling is often denied but can be revealed by performing an interview or through observing facial expressions and behavior. The loss of interest in daily activities manifests itself mostly by a reduced interest in hobbies and being socially withdrawn.

In addition to one of these core symptoms, at least four of the following symptoms are also present: severe changes in appetite that can occur in both directions (by weight increases and losses of more than 5% of body weight in a month); insomnia or excessive sleeping nearly every day; psychomotor changes that cover psychomotor retardation (slowed speech, slower mental activity, and slow movements), or restlessness shown by actions, such as an inability to sit still, plucking at one's clothes, wringing one's hands, and so forth.; fatigue or loss of energy meaning that even routine actions, such as getting washed and dressed require a great deal of effort from the individual; a feeling of worthlessness can be so extreme that the depressed individual blames himself for every setback and suffers from an exaggerated feeling of guilt; impaired concentration and indecisiveness can be prominent with older patients, making it easy to believe that this might be a dementia syndrome, although this diagnosis might not be justified; and finally, thoughts of death, ranging from the conviction that others would be happier without the depressed individual to laying down concrete plans for suicide.

The course taken by a major depressive disorder varies greatly from person to person. After a single episode of major depressive disorder there is a 50% to 60% chance of the occurrence of a second depressive period. If left untreated, a depressive episode can last from a minimum of six months to as long as several years [25].

Dysthymic disorder is a milder form of depression that causes psychologic, physical, and social functions to be hampered but to a lesser degree than with major depressive disorder. The diagnosis is made if a depressive state of mind is present for most of the day, for more days than not, over a period of two years. At least two of the following symptoms must occur: problems with appetite and sleep, low energy levels, low self-image, impaired ability to concentrate or indecisiveness, and feelings of hopelessness [25,49]. Dysthymia is established if no major depressive disorder was experienced over a period of two years. If such a disorder was experienced, then this is known as a chronic major depressive disorder. A major depressive disorder still may occur after experiencing a two-year dysthymic disorder [25].

"Depression not otherwise specified" covers depressive symptoms that do not satisfy the diagnosis of major depressive disorder, dysthymia, or other assorted syndromes (eg, bipolar disorder, manic depression). Minor depressive disorder, also known as subsyndromal depression, is an example. Only two to four of the previous mentioned nine symptoms of major depressive disorder are present with subsyndromal depression and these are present for at least two weeks [25]. The subsyndromal form occurs in the elderly more frequently than major depressive disorder and is likewise associated with functional deterioration, psychosocial disability, and an increased likelihood of experiencing a major depressive disorder [45,52].

Depressive complaints in an older patient can be overshadowed by problems of a somatic nature, a so-called "somatically masked depression." The underlying depression, in these cases, is masked by vague physical complaints, such as fatigue, feelings of faintness, backache, and abdominal pain, and other complaints. The reasons for this somatization of complaints is the taboo surrounding any appearance of being "mentally ill," often a consideration for older patients [51]. This taboo can prevent older patients from expressing their feelings of depression. In addition to this, older patients are more used to expressing physical ailments than talking about psychologic suffering.

In the case of depressive-pseudodementia, it is often difficult to distinguish between incipient dementia and a depressive syndrome causing cognitive dysfunction (loss of interest, difficulty in concentrating, memory defects, and so on). These disorders can be present to such a degree that the criteria for dementia are apparently satisfied leading to an incorrect diagnosis being made [25,49,51]. The characteristics of the cognitive disorders at the beginning of the illness allow us to distinguish between the two [51]. In older patients suffering from depression, the cognitive disorder develops subacutely (over weeks) while in patients suffering from dementia, it develops more slowly and insidiously (over months). The ability of older patients who develop depressive-pseudodementia to take care of themselves is reduced. Patients who experience depression find their thought processes are slower, older patients who experience dementia find this is sometimes accelerated and thinking is often characterized by a certain amount of verbosity. Attention span often is reduced with depression, but generally well-preserved in older patients who develop dementia. In older patients who have depression, short-term and long-term memory seem to be equally severely disturbed, in contrast to findings relating to older patients who experience dementia, where short-term memory is noticeably more disturbed [51]. Dementia, especially in its initial phase, has a significant degree of comorbidity with depression [53,54].

An elderly depressed patient can also display other symptoms, such as restlessness and anxiety, hypochondria or paranoia (psychotic depression). These psychotic symptoms can prompt the erroneous consideration of other psychiatric disorders, such as late onset schizophrenia [51].

Risk Factors

Heredity plays an important part in the development of depression [55,56]. Depression also can arise as a side effect of certain types of drugs (analgesics, antihypertensive agents, anti-Parkinson's agents, steroids). Illnesses, such as a cerebrovascular accident, cancer, dementia, diabetes mellitus, lower back/ neck pain and other diseases, causing functional impediments also can lead to an increased risk for depression in older patients [55].

In addition to these biological factors, psychosocial risk factors also exist. Depression can develop in older patients as a result of an unexpected life event, chronic stress, low socio-economic status, or a low personal assessment of one's actual prospects. Furthermore, women, unmarried individuals, widows, and widowers form a significant risk group [55–57]. Starting to live in a residential setting or the effects of a stay in hospital with the possible experience of pain, accompanying sensory deprivation, and immobilization can increase the likelihood of developing depression [58]. A recent cross-sectional study showed that a history of previous depression, bereavement in the previous year, premorbid disability, cognitive impairment, and poor perceived psychosocial supports characterize older medical inpatients at particularly high risk for depression [44].

The presence of different risk factors simultaneously can increase the chances of developing depression. The effects are influenced moreover by the absence or presence of a good social network [43,46,56].

Cognitive Assessment

The Yale Task Force on Geriatric Assessment recommends to use a single question, "Do you often feel sad or depressed?" as a first screening for depression in older persons [59]. The adverb "often" is intended to differentiate depression from normal fluctuations in mood [60]. Although this single question has a high positive predictive value and a high specificity for depression, its sensitivity is low, probably because the elderly are less inclined to admit feelings of sadness [59]; therefore, this simple question can serve as an introduction to a more detailed investigation.

The Geriatric Depression Scale (GDS) is the most widely used and the most reliable and valid scale for screening depression in older adults [55,61]. It is mainly used as a screening instrument whereby the diagnosis of depression only can be made following an extensive psychiatric interview. The GDS also can be used as an intensity record (severity of the depression) or to measure the effects of the treatment. The GDS is a self-assessment scale consisting of 30 items. This instrument can also be used in the form of an interview. This method is especially worthwhile when dealing with elderly hospitalized patients and elderly patients who experience reduced cognitive ability. Given that the GDS consists exclusively of psychologic items, confusion between depression and somatic complaints (to be attributed to physical disorders) are avoided [51]. The total GDS score varies from 0 to 30, where scores from 0 to 10 indicate a normal state of mind, 11 to 20 indicate mild depression, and 21 to 30 indicate severe depression [62]. Initially, a cut-off score of 11 was taken as a benchmark for the presence of depression, later a cut-off score of 14 was introduced for the detection of depression in older patients who have somatic illnesses. Various abridged versions of the GDS have been developed, such as the GDS 15-item and the GDS 10-item version. The diagnostic value of these shorter forms is comparable to the GDS 30-item version [63–65]. Also the GDS 5-item and a GDS 4-item scale are found to be reliable shorter versions [65–67]; however, they are mainly recommended as a first screening for older hospitalized patients or for patients who have dementia, given that these patients become tired quickly and have a limited ability to concentrate. Furthermore, a GDS 12-item version has been developed suitable for older people living in nursing and residential care settings [68].

The GDS, however, is not used often by care providers because of the difficult and sensitive questions that they have to ask the patient or because of the refusal of older patients to cooperate with inquiries regarding their psychologic condition [69]. For this reason, Hammond and colleagues [70] developed a new 6-item instrument where assessment takes place on the basis of observations by medical staff during day-to-day care. Observation scales also contribute more to the screening of depression in older adults with communicative disorders, such as those suffering from cerebrovascular disorders, those who are deaf, or those who have cognitive disorders. Although further research is necessary in the use of this instrument, the first results are promising.

Another instrument that might be used in demented patients is the Cornell Scale for Depression in Dementia (CSDD) [71]. This 19-item clinician-administered checklist uses information from patients and primary caregivers. When compared with other scales, the CSDD has been found to be the best diagnostic scale for detecting depression in dementia in two recent studies [59,72]. Diagnosing depression in dementia, however, becomes increasingly difficult as dementia advances, which is reflected in the higher optimal cut-off values on CSDD as one moves from mild dementia (CSDD cut-off score of 7) to moderate-severe dementia (CSDD cut-off score of 13) [59].

DELIRIUM
Epidemiology
Delirium is a prevalent disorder; estimates range from 14% to 80% of all elderly patients hospitalized for the treatment of acute physical illness experience an episode of delirium [73–75]. The marked variability in the epidemiology of delirium results from the differences in study populations, diagnostic criteria, and case-finding and research techniques [75,76]. Moreover, delirium has been shown to contribute independently to poor outcomes of acute care [74,77–79]. Delirious patients experience greater in-hospital functional decline compared with nondelirious patients [74,79]. Because of their inability to think clearly, delirious patients are unable to care for themselves. They frequently exhibit unsafe behaviors that require a greater intensity of nursing care [80,81] and, more frequently, result in the use of physical restraints [82,83]. The length of hospitalization is significantly longer for delirious patients than for nondelirious patients, even after adjustments for severity of illness and DRG classification are made [79,84]. Hospital mortality rates are higher,

ranging from 10% to 65% [74], in which the lower rates of mortality are probably attributable to milder forms of delirium [78].

Clinical Features

Delirium is a disturbance of consciousness with reduced ability to focus, sustain, or shift attention, and a change in cognition or the development of a perceptual disturbance that occurs over a short period of time and fluctuates over the course of the day [25]. Historically, delirium has been differentiated from other cognitive disorders, such as dementia, on the basis of its acute onset and transient and fluctuating course. Yet, because the frequent coexistence of delirium with dementia and depression, this is not accomplished so easily clinically, the clinical features of delirium, dementia, and depression are compared in Table 1.

Table 1			
A comparison of the clinical features of delirium, dementia, and depression			
Clinical feature	Delirium	Dementia	Depression
Onset	Sudden/abrupt	Insidious/slow, usually unrecognized	Variable
Course	Short with diurnal fluctuations in symptomatology	Chronic and progressive	Variable, symptoms typically worse in the early morning
Progression	Abrupt	Protracted	Variable
Consciousness	Altered	Clear except in severe cases	Clear
Attention	Impaired; fluctuates	Initially normal	Generally normal
Orientation	Generally impaired, severity varies	Generally normal[a]	Selective disorientation
Memory	Recent and immediate impaired	Recent and remote impaired	Selective impairment
Thinking	Disorganized, incoherent	Difficulty with abstraction, thoughts impoverished	Intact with themes of hopelessness and helplessness
Perception	Misperceptions common with illusions, hallucinations and delusions	Misperceptions usually absent	Intact
Psychomotor behavior	Variable: hypokinetic, hyperkinetic, and mixed	Generally normal	Variable
Assessment	Distracted from task; numerous errors	Struggles with assessment to find appropriate reply	Generally lacks motivations, frequent "don't know" answers

[a]Orientation can be impaired (eg., vascular dementia or advanced stage of dementia).

From Milisen K, Steeman E, Foreman MD. Early detection and prevention of delirium in older patients with cancer. Eur J Cancer Care 2004;13:494–500; with permission.

Although generally considered to be reversible with complete recovery, recent studies [85,86] have shown symptoms of delirium to persist for many months beyond the initial episode of delirium, and others [87] have documented sustained and significant loss of memory and higher cognitive functions with an increased risk for dementia.

Delirious patients exhibit a wide range of behaviors, complicating the process of making a diagnosis and planning interventions. Although specific etiologies have not been linked with different subtypes of patterns of delirium, it is speculated that the variation is a function of etiology [88]. Lipowski [88] identified three variants of delirium based on verbal and nonverbal behaviors exhibited by the patient. These variants are called hyperactive, hypoactive, or mixed. Patients who experience hyperactive delirium exhibit behaviors most commonly recognized as delirium (ie, psychomotor hyperactivity, marked excitability, and a tendency toward hallucinations). Such patients may exhibit hypervigilance, restlessness, fast or loud speech, irritability, combativeness, impatience, swearing, singing, laughing, uncooperativeness, euphoria, anger, wandering, easily starting, distractibility, nightmares, and persistent thoughts [89]. The patient with the hypoactive variant may be lethargic, somnolent, apathetic, and exhibit reduced psychomotor activity, including unawareness, decreased alertness, sparse or slow speech, lethargy, slowed movements, staring, and apathy [89]. This is the "quiet" patient for whom the diagnosis of delirium is often missed. The third variant—mixed—involves behavior that fluctuates between the hyper- and hypoactive variants. In one of the few studies on delirium subtypes, Liptzin and Levkoff [89] required the presence of three or more hyperactive behaviors to be present for the patient to be classified as hyperactive, four or more hypoactive behaviors to diagnose hypoactive, and a positive rating on both types to be considered mixed. Using those criteria with 125 patients diagnosed with delirium, 15% were rated as hyperactive, 19% as hypoactive, 52% had a mixed picture, and 14% had no pattern. The high percentage of mixed behaviors supports the notion of the fluctuating course and partially clarifies the difficulties in recognizing and diagnosing delirium.

The recognition and diagnosis of delirium is complicated significantly when it frequently coexists with other mental disorders [90], most notably dementia and depression, but also with psychotic states to a lesser degree. Delirium has been studied less in patients who have psychiatric disorders [75,91], as these individuals generally are excluded from the study of delirium because of the challenge of recognizing and diagnosing delirium superimposed on a psychotic state [92]. An acute psychosis can mimic a hyperactive delirium; however, the hallucinations experienced by psychotic patients tend to be more systematic, bizarre, and typically auditory versus visual for delirious patients. Differential diagnosis is facilitated by knowing the psychiatric history of the individual [92].

Finally, anxiety can mimic hyperactive delirium [93]. Anxiety is common among hospitalized older patients resulting from physical discomforts, unfamiliarity of the hospital environment and procedures, separation from family, and a subjective cognitive appraisal of the event as threatening. Although it is critical to differentiate anxiety from delirium, evidence linking anxiety to the genesis of delirium is inconclusive [93,94].

Risk Factors

A current and prevalent model of risk for delirium was offered by Inouye and colleagues [95,96]. In this model, delirium results from the interaction between an individual's baseline vulnerability, or predisposing risk for delirium, and precipitating factors or events. Baseline vulnerability arises from increased age, existing cognitive impairment (eg, dementia and depression), sensory impairments, inactivity, and comorbidity or severity of illness–the greater the number of vulnerabilities the greater the risk for delirium. Within the context of a vulnerable individual, certain factors can precipitate an episode of delirium. In general, these factors include: dehydration, malnutrition, immobility, psychoactive medications, and disorienting environmental factors. To some extent these precipitating factors vary across patient populations. For example, although not important for medical patients, hypoxia intraoperative blood loss and poorly managed pain are important for surgical patients [97,98]. For terminally ill patients, dehydration and opioid toxicity are known precipitating factors [99,100]. In any patient population, however, risk is dynamic and, therefore, must be continually re-evaluated over time.

Cognitive Assessment

Most recommended procedures for the assessment of delirium consist of a series of instruments: a brief general cognitive screen, a diagnostic tool, and a measure of severity [90]. Usually, the assessment procedure begins with a general cognitive bedside screening instrument such as the MMSE (Mini-Mental State Examination) [34], or the SPMSQ (Short Portable Mental Status Questionnaire) [101]. Instruments such as these provide information by which one can answer the question, "Is there evidence that this patient is cognitively impaired?" Although these instruments are generally brief and easy to use, they can impose undue demands on the patient, and these instruments tend to have strong educational and language biases [102].

To counter these criticisms, instruments using information from everyday nurse-patient interactions have been developed. The NEECHAM Confusion Scale [103], and the DOS Scale (Delirium Observation Screening Scale) [104] are two such instruments. If the use of any one of these instruments produces evidence that the patient is cognitively impaired, then it is recommended that further evaluation of the patient include a diagnostic tool. The most frequently used tool for the diagnosis of delirium is the CAM (Confusion Assessment Method) [105]. A major criticism of the CAM has been the inability to use it with patients who cannot verbally communicate (eg, those undergoing mechanical ventilation). Ely and colleagues [106], however, recently modified the CAM to be valid and reliable with such patients. This version has been named the CAM-ICU. After determining that the cognitive impairment is the result of the patient's being delirious, it may be useful to determine its severity. Again, several acceptable instruments exist, notably the DRS (Delirium Rating Scale) [107], the CSE (Confusional State Evaluation) [108], and the DI [109,110]. In particular, the DRS represents a significant advance over other symptom-rating scales used to detect delirium. The criteria for delirium have been operational-ized, thereby providing information on cognitive and behavioral symptoms. The DRS was revised recently, becoming the DRS-Revised-98 (DRS-R-98) [111]. Advantages of the revised scale include its ability to provide information about severity over a broad range of symptoms and to be a useful diagnostic and assessment tool for longitudinal studies.

More in-depth reviews of these instruments and others can be found else-where [90,102,112,113].

SUMMARY

Today, older people live longer. In the United States a 70-year-old person can expect to live another 14.7 years [114]. In Europe, the life expectancy at the age of 65 for men and women is on average 16 and 19 years, respectively [115]. Consequently, these individuals are more likely to be confronted and have to deal with an alteration in their cognitive functioning; however, to deal effec-tively and appropriately with this decline, it must be determined whether or not the decline is a benign consequence of aging or the result of a serious health problem. In this article, "cognitive decline" was clarified from a benign and ge-neric label to one consisting of various types of impairments each with its spe-cific representation, characteristics, and implications for care. As a result, failing to assess the cognitive abilities of an older individual should be unacceptable, unprofessional practice, and may even be considered professional neglect. At worst, failing to assess an older person's cognitive abilities contributes to inef-fective and inappropriate care and treatment while relatives or significant others may be wrongly informed about the individual's prognosis (eg, the pos-sible (ir)reversibility of the disorder). The older person easily is labeled "con-fused", "depressed," or "demented" without sound evidence to support this. Moreover, such labels profoundly influence how others interact with these peo-ple. At the least, many consider these people incompetent, and such labels are infrequently removed.

Nurses play a pivotal role in the recognition, diagnosis, and prevention and care of cognitive decline in older people. Because nurses have significant, more frequent, and more continuous contact with older persons, and their relatives, nurses are the obvious person to gather and compare relevant details about the older person's cognitive and social functioning (eg, at home versus inhospital behavior); this can be easily accomplished using the informal, naturally occur-ring method of assessment discussed earlier. Furthermore, when integrating structured assessment into routine care, nurses can identify minor impairments easily and earlier and as a result have the potential to prevent or promptly re-verse the impairment in cognitive functioning. To enable nurses to accomplish this, this article provides a description of the diagnostic dilemmas of dementia, depression, and delirium in the elderly along with current recommendations for the standardized assessment and systematic monitoring of cognition.

Acknowledgments

Shari Walczak (The Pennsylvania State University) for assistance with manuscript preparation.

References

[1] Foreman MD, Fletcher K, Mion LC, et al. Assessing cognitive function. In: Mezey MD, Fulmer T, Abraham I, editors. Geriatric nursing protocols for best practice. 2nd edition. New York: Springer Pub. Co.; 2003. p. 99–115.

[2] Dellasega C. Assessment of cognition in the elderly. Nurs Clin North Am 1998;33(3): 395–405.

[3] Williams MP, Salisbury SA. Cognitive assessment. In: Stone JT, Wyman JF, Salisbury SA, editors. Clinical gerontological nursing: a guide to advanced practice. 2nd edition. Philadelphia: WB Saunders; 1999. p. 129–54.

[4] Tagliareni E, Waters V. The ageing experience. In: Anderson MA, Braun JV, editors. Caring for the elderly client. 2nd edition. Philadelphia: F.A. Davis Company; 1999. p. 3–25.

[5] Lang M. Screening for cognitive impairment in the older adult. Nurse Pract 2001;26(11): 26–41.

[6] Lekan-Rutledge D. Functional assessment. In: Matteson MA, McConnel ES, Linton AD, editors. Gerontological nursing: concepts and practice. 2nd edition. Philadelphia: WB Saunders; 1997. p. 67–111.

[7] Smith M, Breithart W, Platt M. A critique of instruments and methods to detect, diagnose, and rate delirium. J Pain Symptom Manage 1995;10(1):35–77.

[8] Greenhalgh T. How to read a paper. Papers that report diagnostic or screening tests. BMJ 1997;315:540–3.

[9] Engberg SJ, McDowell J. Comprehensive geriatric assessment. In: Stone JT, Wyman JF, Salisbury SA, editors. Clinical gerontological nursing: a guide to advanced practice. 2nd edition. Philadelphia: WB Saunders; 1999. p. 63–85.

[10] Evans DA, Funkenstein HH, Albert MS, et al. Prevalence of Alzheimer's disease in a community population of older persons: higher than previously reported. JAMA 1989;262: 2551–6.

[11] US Department of Health and Human Services. National Institutes of Health. Alzheimer's disease: unraveling the mystery. Washington, DC: US Department of Health and Human Services; 2002. Publication 01–3782.

[12] Hofman A, Rocca WA, Brayne C, et al. The prevalence of dementia in Europe: a collaborative study of 1980–1990 findings. Int J Epidemiol 1991;20(3):736–48.

[13] Berr C, Wancata J, Ritchie K. Prevalence of dementia in the elderly in Europe. Eur Neuropsychopharmacol 2005;15(4):463–71.

[14] Hoyert DL, Kung HC, Smith BL. Deaths: preliminary data for 2003. Natl Vital Stat Rep 2005;53:1–48.

[15] Fick D, Foreman M. Consequences of not recognizing delirium superimposed on dementia in hospitalized elderly individuals. J Gerontol Nurs 2000;26:30–40.

[16] Fick DM, Agostini JV, Inouye SK. Delirium superimposed on dementia: a systematic review. J Am Geriatr Soc 2002;50:1723–32.

[17] Fick D, Kolanowski A, Waller JL, et al. Delirium superimposed on dementia in a community-living managed care population: a three year retrospective study of prevalence, costs, and utilization. J Gerontol A Biol Sci Med Sci 2005;60(6):748–53.

[18] Aalten P, de Vugt ME, Jaspers N, et al. The course of neuropsychiatric symptoms in dementia. Part I: findings from the two-year longitudinal Maasbed study. Int J Geriatr Psychiatry 2005;20(6):523–30.

[19] Dal Forno G, Palermo MT, Donohue JE, et al. Depressive symptoms, sex, and risk for Alzheimer's disease. Ann Neurol 2005;57(3):381–7.

[20] Harrow BS, Mahoney DF, Mendelsohn AB, et al. Variation in cost of informal caregiving and formal-service use for people with Alzheimer's disease. Am J Alzheimers Dis Other Demen 2004;19:299–308.

[21] Bloom BS, de Pouvourville N, Straus WL. Cost of illness of Alzheimer's disease: how useful are current estimates? Gerontologist 2003;43(2):158–64.

[22] Koppel R. Alzheimer's disease: the cost to US businesses in 2002. Chicago: Alzheimer's Association; 2002.

[23] Jönsson L, Berr C. Cost of dementia in Europe. Eur J Neurol 2005;12(Suppl 1):50–3.

[24] McKhann G, Drachman D, Folstein M, et al. Clinical diagnosis of Alzheimer's disease: report of the NINCDS-ADRDA Work Group under the auspices of Department of Health and Human Services Task Force on Alzheimer's Disease. Neurology 1984;34:939–44.

[25] American Psychiatric Association. Diagnostic and statistical manual of mental disorders. 4th edition. Washington, DC: American Psychiatric Association; 2000. p. 135–158, 345–428.

[26] Petersen RC, Smith GE, Waring SC, et al. Mild cognitive impairment: clinical characterization and outcome. Arch Neurol 1999;56:303–8.

[27] Carlsson C, Gleason C, Asthana S. Update on diagnosis and treatment of Alzheimer disease. Applied Neurology 2005;1:24–32.

[28] Mosconi L, Tsui WH, De Santi S, et al. Reduced hippocampal metabolism in MCI and AD: automated FDG-PET image analysis. Neurology 2005;64(11):1860–7.

[29] Kukull WA, Higdon R, Bowen JD, et al. Dementia and Alzheimer disease incidence: a prospective cohort study. Arch Neurol 2002;59:1737–46.

[30] Jellinger KA, Attems J. Prevalence and pathogenic role of cerebrovascular lesions in Alzheimer disease. J Neurol Sci 2005;229–230:37–41.

[31] Dufouil C, Richard F, Fievet N, et al. APOE genotype, cholesterol level, lipid-lowering treatment, and dementia: the Three-City Study. Neurology 2005;64:1531–8.

[32] Lott IT, Head E. Alzheimer disease and Down syndrome: factors in pathogenesis. Neurobiol Aging 2005;26:383–9.

[33] Clarfield AM. The reversible dementias: do they reverse? Ann Intern Med 1988;109: 476–86.

[34] Folstein MF, Folstein SE, McHugh PR. "Mini-mental state": a practical method for grading the cognitive state of patients for the clinician. J Psychiatr Res 1975;12:189–98.

[35] Borson S, Scanlan JM, Watanabe J, et al. Simplifying detection of cognitive impairment: comparison of the Mini-Cog and Mini-Mental State Examination in a multiethnic sample. J Am Geriatr Soc 2005;53:871–4.

[36] Buschke H, Kuslansky G, Katz M, et al. Screening for dementia with the memory impairment screen. Neurology 1999;15;52(2):231–8.

[37] Kuslansky G, Buschke H, Katz M, et al. Screening for Alzheimer's disease: the memory impairment screen versus the conventional three-word memory test. J Am Geriatr Soc 2002;50(6):1086–91.

[38] Blessed G, Tomlinson BE, Roth M. The association between quantitative measures of dementia and of senile change in the cerebral grey matter of elderly subjects. Br J Psychiatry 1968;114:797–811.

[39] Hughes CP, Berg L, Danziger WL, et al. A new clinical scale for the staging of dementia. Br J Psychiatry 1982;140:566–72.

[40] Auer S, Reisberg B. The GDS/FAST staging system. Int Psychogeriatr 1997;9:167–71.

[41] Verghese J, Buschke H, Kuslansky G, et al. Antemortem memory impairment screen performance is correlated with postmortem Alzheimer pathology. J Am Geriatr Soc 2003;51(7): 1043–5.

[42] Koenig HG, Meador KG, Cohen HJ, et al. Screening for depression in hospitalized elderly medical patients: taking a closer look. J Am Geriatr Soc 1992;40(10):1013–7.

[43] Jongenelis K, Pot AM, Eisses AM, et al. Prevalence and risk indicators of depression in elderly nursing home patients: the AGED study. J Affect Disord 2004;83(2–3): 135–42.

[44] McCusker J, Cole M, Dufouil C, et al. The prevalence and correlates of major and minor depression in older medical inpatients. J Am Geriatr Soc 2005;53(8):1344–53.

[45] VanItallie TB. Subsyndromal depression in the elderly: underdiagnosed and undertreated. Metabolism 2005;54(5, suppl 1):39–44.

[46] Kurlowicz LH. Social factors and depression in late life. Arch Psychiatr Nurs 1993;7(1): 30–6.

[47] Koenig HG, Meador KG, Cohen HJ, et al. Self-rated depression scales and screening for major depression in the older hospitalized patient with medical illness. J Am Geriatr Soc 1988;36(8):699–706.

[48] Koenig HG, Shelp F, Goli V. Survival and health care utilization in elderly medical inpatients with major depression. J Am Geriatr Soc 1989;37(7):599–606.

[49] Zisook S. Depression in late life. Diagnosis, course, and consequences. Postgrad Med 1996;100(4):143–56.

[50] Agrell B, Dehlin O. Comparison of six depression rating scales in geriatric stroke patients. Stroke 1989;20(9):1190–4.

[51] Godderis J, Van de Ven L, Wils V. Stemmingsstoornissen bij ouder wordenden. In: Handboek geriatrische psychiatrie. Leuven/Apeldoorn, (Belgium): Garant; 1992. p. 268–318.

[52] Koenig HG, Meador KG, Shelp F, et al. Major depressive order in hospitalized medically ill patients: an examination of young and elderly male veterans. J Am Geriatr Soc 1991;39(9):881–90.

[53] Foresell Y, Winblad B. Major depression in a population of demented and nondemented older people: prevalence and correlates. J Am Geriatr Soc 1998;46(1):27–30.

[54] Vilalta-Franch J, Lopez-Pousa S, Llinas-Regla J. Prevalence of depressive disorders in dementia. Rev Neurol 1998;26(149):57–60.

[55] Kurlowicz LH. Niche Faculty. Depression in elderly patients. In: Abraham I, Bottrell MM, Fulmer T, editors. Geriatric nursing protocols for best practice. New York: Springer Pub. Co.; 1999. p. 111–30.

[56] Heun R, Hein S. Risk factors of major depression in the elderly. Eur Psychiatry 2005;20(3): 199–204.

[57] Dreyfus JK. Depression assessment and interventions in the medically ill frail elderly. J Gerontol Nurs 1988;14(9):27–36.

[58] Beck DA, Koenig HG, Beck JS. Depression. Clin Geriatr Med 1998;14(4):765–86.

[59] Lam CK, Lim PP, Low BL, et al. Depression in dementia: a comparative and validation study of four brief scales in the elderly Chinese. Int J Geriatr Psychiatry 2004;19(5):422–8.

[60] Lachs MS, Feinstein AR, Cooney LM Jr, et al. A simple procedure for general screening for functional disability in elderly patients. Ann Intern Med 1990;112(9):699–706.

[61] Brink TL, Yesavage JA, Lum O, et al. Screening tests for geriatric depression. Clin Gerontol 1982;1:37–41.

[62] Abraham IL, Wofford AB, Lichtenberg PA, et al. Factor structure of the geriatric depression scale in a cohort of depressed nursing home residents. Int J Geriatr Psychiatry 1994;9(7): 611–7.

[63] Burke WJ, Roccaforte WH, Wengel SP. The short form of the geriatric depression scale: a comparison with the 30-item form. J Geriatr Psychiatry Neurol 1991;4:173–8.

[64] de Craen AJ, Heeren TJ, Gussekloo J. Accuracy of the 15-item geriatric depression scale (GDS-15) in a community sample of the oldest old. Int J Geriatr Psychiatry 2003;18(1): 63–6.

[65] D'Ath P, Katona P, Mullan E, et al. Screening, detection and management of depression in elderly primary care attenders. I: the acceptability and performance of the 15 Item Geriatric Depression Scale (GDS 15) and the development of short versions. Fam Pract 1994;11(3):260–6.

[66] van Marwijk HW, Wallace P, de Bock GH, et al. Evaluation of the feasibility, reliability and diagnostic value of shortened versions of the geriatric depression scale. Br J Gen Pract 1995;45(393):195–9.

[67] Weeks SK, McGann PE, Michaels TK, et al. Comparing various short-form Geriatric Depression Scales leads to the GDS-5/15. J Nurs Scholarsh 2003;35(2):133–7.

[68] Sutcliffe C, Cordingley L, Burns A, et al. A new version of the geriatric depression scale for nursing and residential home populations: the geriatric depression scale (residential) (GDS-12R). Int Psychogeriatr 2000;12(2):173–81.

[69] Hammond MF. Doctors' and nurses' observations on the Geriatric Depression Rating Scale. Age Ageing 2004;33(2):189–92.

[70] Hammond MF, O'Keeffe ST, Barer DH. Development and validation of a brief observer-rated screening scale for depression in elderly medical patients. Age Ageing 2000;29: 511–5.

[71] Alexopoulos GS, Abrams RC, Young RC, et al. Cornell scale for depression in dementia. Biol Psychiatry 1988;23(3):271–84.

[72] Muller-Thomsen T, Arlt S, Mann U, et al. Detecting depression in Alzheimer's disease: evaluation of four different scales. Arch Clin Neuropsychol 2005;20(2):271–6.

[73] Foreman MD. Acute confusion in the elderly. Annu Rev Nurs Res 1993;11:3–30.

[74] Inouye SK, Rusing JT, Foreman MD, et al. Does delirium contribute to poor hospital outcomes? A three-site epidemiologic study. J Gen Intern Med 1998;13:234–42.

[75] Lindesay J, Rockwood K, Rolfson D. The epidemiology of delirium. In: Lindesay J, Rockwood K, Macdonald A, editors. Delirium in old age. Oxford (UK): Oxford University Press; 2002. p. 27–50.

[76] Milisen K, Foreman MD, Godderis J, et al. Delirium in the elderly: nursing assessment and management. Nurs Clin North Am 1998;33:417–39.

[77] Francis J, Kapoor WN. Prognosis after hospital discharge of older medical patients with delirium. J Am Geriatr Soc 1992;40:601–6.

[78] O'Keefe SO, Lavan J. The prognostic significance of delirium in older hospital patients. J Am Geriatr Soc 1997;45:174–8.

[79] Pompei P, Foreman MD, Rudberg MA, et al. Delirium in hospitalized older persons: outcomes and predictors. J Am Geriatr Soc 1994;42:809–15.

[80] Brannstrom B, Gusatafson Y, Norberg A, et al. Problems of basic nursing care in acutely confused and non-confused hip-fracture patients. Scand J Caring Sci 1989;3(1):27–34.

[81] Francis J, Hilko E, Kapoor WN. Older patients with delirium: intensity of hospital resource use. J Gen Intern Med 1994;9(Suppl. 2):43.

[82] Ludwick R. Clinical decision making: recognition of confusion and application of restraints. Orthop Nurs 1999;18(1):65–72.

[83] Sullivan-Marx EM. Delirium and physical restraint in the hospitalized elderly. Image J Nurs Sch 1994;26:295–300.

[84] Francis J, Strong S, Martin D, et al. Manifestations and outcomes of delirium in elderly patients. Clin Res 1989;37:311A.

[85] Levkoff SE, Yang FM, Liptzin B. Delirium: the importance of subsyndromal states. Primary Psychiatry 2004;11(11):40–4.

[86] Rockwood K, Cosway S, Carver D, et al. The risk of dementia and death after delirium. Age Ageing 1999;28(6):551–6.

[87] Jackson JC, Gordon SM, Hart RP, et al. The association between delirium and cognitive decline: a review of the empirical literature. Neuropsychol Rev 2004;14:87–98.

[88] Lipowski ZJ. Transient cognitive disorders (delirium/acute confusional states) in the elderly. Am J Psychiatry 1983;140:1426–36.

[89] Liptzin B, Levkoff SE. An empirical study of delirium subtypes. Br J Psychiatry 1992;161: 843–5.

[90] Robertsson B. The instrumentation of delirium. In: Lindesay J, Rockwood K, Macdonald A, editors. Delirium in old age. Oxford (UK): Oxford University Press; 2002. p. 9–25.

[91] Huang SC, Tsai SJ, Chan CH, et al. Characteristics and outcome of delirium in psychiatric inpatients. Psychiatry Clin Neurosci 1998;52:47–50.

[92] Caraceni A, Grassi L. Delirium: acute confusional states in palliative medicine. Oxford (UK): Oxford University Press; 2003.

[93] Misra S, Ganzini L. Delirium, depression, and anxiety. Crit Care Clin 2003;19:771–87.

[94] Kress JP, Hall JB. Delirium and sedation. Crit Care Clin 2004;20:419–33.

[95] Inouye SK, Viscoli CM, Horwitz RI, et al. A predictive model for delirium in hospitalized medical patients based on admission characteristics. Ann Intern Med 1993;119: 474–81.

[96] Inouye SK, Charpentier PA. Precipitating factors for delirium in hospitalized elderly persons. Predictive model and interrelationship with baseline vulnerability. JAMA 1996; 275:852–7.

[97] Bohner H, Hummel TC, Habel U, et al. Predicting delirium after vascular surgery: a model based on pre- and intraoperative data. Ann Surg 2003;238(1):149–56.

[98] Milisen K, Foreman MD, Abraham IL, et al. A nurse-led interdisciplinary intervention program for delirium in elderly hip-fracture patients. J Am Geriatr Soc 2001;49(5): 523–32.

[99] Breitbart W, Marotta R, Platt MM, et al. A double-blind trial of haloperidol, chlorpromazine, and lorazepam for the treatment of delirium in hospitalized AIDS patients. Am J Psychiatry 1996;153(2):231–7.

[100] Milisen K, Steeman E, Foreman MD. Early detection and prevention of delirium in older patients with cancer. Eur J Cancer Care (UK) 2004;13:494–500.

[101] Pfeiffer E. A short portable mental status questionnaire for the assessment of organic brain deficit in elderly patients. J Am Geriatr Soc 1975;23:433–41.

[102] Foreman MD, Vermeersch PEH. Measuring cognitive status. In: Frank-Stromborg M, Olsen SJ, editors. Instruments for clinical health care research. 3rd edition. Sudbury (MA): Jones and Bartlett; 2004. p. 100–27.

[103] Neelon VJ, Champagne MT, Carlsson JR, et al. The NEECHAM Confusion Scale: construction, validation, and clinical testing. Nurs Res 1996;45:324–30.

[104] Schuurmans MJ, Shortridge-Baggett LM, Duursma SA. The Delirium Observation Screening Scale: a screening instrument for delirium. Res Theory Nurs Pract 2003;17(1): 31–50.

[105] Inouye SK, van Dyck CH, Alessi CA, et al. Clarifying confusion: the Confusion Assessment Method. A new method for detection of delirium. Ann Intern Med 1990;113:941–8.

[106] Ely EW, Inouye SK, Bernard GR, et al. Delirium in mechanically ventilated patients. Validity and reliability of the Confusion Assessment Method for the intensive care unit (CAM-ICU). JAMA 2001;286(21):2703–10.

[107] Trzepacz PT, Baker RW, Greenhouse J. A symptom rating scale for delirium. Psychiatry Res 1988;23:89–97.

[108] Robertsson B, Karlsson I, Styrud E, et al. Confusional State Evaluation (CSE): an instrument for measuring severity of delirium in the elderly. Br J Psychiatry 1997;170:565–70.

[109] McCusker J, Cole M, Bellavance F, et al. Reliability and validity of a new measure of severity of delirium. Int Psychogeriatr 1998;10:421–33.

[110] McCusker J, Cole MG, Dendukuri N, et al. The delirium index, a measure of the severity of delirium: new findings on reliability, validity, and responsiveness. J Am Geriatr Soc 2004;52(10):1744–9.

[111] Trzepacz PT, Mittal D, Torres R, et al. Validations of the delirium rating scale-revised-98: comparison with the delirium rating scale and the cognitive test for delirium. J Neuropsychiatry Clin Neurosci 2001;13(2):229–42.

[112] Rapp CG, Wakefield B, Kundrat M, et al. Acute confusion assessment instruments: clinical versus research usability. Appl Nurs Res 2000;13:37–45.

[113] Schuurmans MJ, Deschamps PI, Markham SW, et al. The measurement of delirium: review of scales. Res Theory Nurs Pract 2003;17(3):207–24.

[114] Arias E. United States life tables, 2002. National vital statistics reports, vol 53, no 6. Hyattsville (MD): National Center for Health Statistics. 2004. Available at: www.cdc.gov/nchs/data/nvsr/nvsr53/nvsr53_06.pdf. Accessed July 27, 2005.

[115] Eurostat Yearbook 2003. Office for Official Publications of the EU, Luxembourg. Eurostat: statistical yearbook on candidate countries 2003. Available at: http://www.eurofound.eu.int/areas/qualityoflife/eurlife/index.php?template=3&radioindic=2&idDomain=1. Accessed Retrieved on July 27, 2005.

Nurs Clin N Am 41 (2006) 23–41

NURSING CLINICS
OF NORTH AMERICA

ELSEVIER
SAUNDERS

Assessment of Psychoemotional and Behavioral Status in Patients with Dementia

Lisa L. Onega, PhD, RN, FNP, CNS, GNP

School of Nursing, Radford University, P.O. Box 6964, 501 Stockton Street, Radford, VA 24142, USA

DEPRESSION IN OLDER ADULTS

Approximately 50% of older adults who develop dementia have minor depressive disorder or depressive symptoms that interfere with functioning and 15% to 20% have major depressive disorder [1–3]. Some features of depression that may be more commonly present in older adults than in younger adults are agitation, hypochondriasis, loneliness, retardation, somatic symptoms or altered sleep and appetite, and suicidal ideation. Older adults often do not report symptoms of depression, and symptoms vary a great deal from one older adult to another. Thus, even for experienced clinicians identification of depression in this population can be challenging [1,2,4]. Depression is associated with poor outcomes in older adults, including high rates of hospitalization, nursing home admissions, morbidity, and mortality and cognitive decline in older adults with dementia [1–6]. Key components of depression in older adults, instrumentation as an adjunct to clinical evaluation, assessment of depression in nursing homes, individualized care for older adults with dementia who are depressed, behavioral assessment, and issues related to psychoemotional and behavioral status are discussed.

KEY COMPONENTS OF DEPRESSION IN OLDER ADULTS

Research has focused primarily on the neurologic and physical factors related to depression in dementia; however, understanding depression in the context of older adults' lives enables clinicians to assess individuals' depressive symptoms comprehensively and implement treatment targeting these symptoms. When assessing older adults who experience dementia for depression, nurses need to identify coping strategies, developmental issues that older adults may be experiencing, the meaning that individuals give to an event, physical and psychologic resources, situational factors that may be exacerbating

E-mail address: lonega@radford.edu

0029-6465/06/$ – see front matter
doi:10.1016/j.cnur.2005.09.003

depression, social support, socioeconomic issues that are related to emotional health, and stressors. Additionally, clinicians should take note of experiences resulting in significant loss or perceived threats that last longer than a week as these may be associated with depression in older adults who experience dementia [6].

Zubenko and colleagues [3] examined 243 individuals with probable Alzheimer's disease and 151 cognitively intact older adults to understand the clinical features of depression in older adults with Alzheimer's disease. They found that when a major depressive disorder was diagnosed, older adults with Alzheimer's disease and cognitively intact older adults had approximately the same number of total symptoms; however, individuals with Alzheimer's disease were more likely to have decreased concentration and indecisiveness and less likely to have sleep impairment, feelings of worthlessness, and guilt than cognitively intact individuals. Other symptoms that were more common in older adults with Alzheimer's disease than in cognitively intact individuals were psychomotor agitation, retardation, fatigue, and loss of energy. The clinical features of major depression were similar among individuals with mild, moderate, and severe Alzheimer's disease who were depressed, indicating that severity of dementia did not influence the presentation of depressive symptoms. The researchers suggest that older adults with Alzheimer's disease may have a common depressive symptom profile.

Between 22.5% and 54.4% of individuals with dementia are depressed; therefore, understanding the depressive syndrome of Alzheimer's disease and identifying treatments best suited to the symptoms presented is needed [7]. To comprehensively identify depressive symptoms in older adults and design treatments that match symptoms, in 2004 Onega evaluated the content validity of the Depressive Symptom Assessment for Older Adults with seven older adults. The content validation portion of the study was done in two phases. In phase one, interviews with older adults ranged from 1 hour and 15 minutes to 3 hours and 30 minutes with the average interview lasting 2 hours and 12 minutes. Content validation was determined based on percent agreement amongst older adults [8]. The Depressive Symptom Assessment for Older Adults was revised using the older adults' feedback. In phase two, interviews with older adults ranged from 1 hour to 2 hours and 30 minutes with an average of 1 hour and 20 minutes. Again, the instrument was modified based on the older adults' comments. Older adults received $50 for participation in each phase of the study. Twenty-seven depressive symptom items were included in the instrument and divided into six categories or subscales with two to six items in each subscale. Four response options are possible for each of the 27 items: none, mild, moderate, and severe. Total scores for the Depressive Symptom Assessment for Older Adults range from 0, indicating no depression, to 81, indicating the most severe depression. Scores are also obtained on each of the six subscales. If significant symptoms are present in a certain subscale, interventions targeting that group of symptoms can be instituted (Table 1). Each category of symptoms is discussed below.

Table 1	
Subscales and items on the depressive symptom assessment for older adults	
Subscales	Items
Subscale 1: Melancholic behavior	1. Depressed appearance or behavior
	2. Worthlessness
	3. Inability to experience enjoyment
	4. Decreased work and interest
	5. Retardation
Score range for Subscale 1: 0–18	6. Little energy
Subscale 2: Disagreeable behavior	7. Irritability
	8. Physical agitation
	9. Loss of insight
	10. Decreased awareness of emotional state
Score range for Subscale 2: 0–15	11. Decreased emotional responsiveness
Subscale 3: Anxiety	12. Psychological anxiety
	13. Somatic anxiety
	14. Hypochondriasis
Score range for Subscale 3: 0–12	15. Guilt feelings
Subscale 4: Sleep impairment	16. Initial insomnia
	17. Middle insomnia
	18. Delayed insomnia
Score range for Subscale 4: 0–12	19. Daytime drowsiness
Subscale 5: Appetite impairment	20. Change in appetite
Score range for Subscale 5: 0–6	21. Weight change
Subscale 6: Lack of meaning in life	22. Hopelessness
	23. Suicide
	24. Lack of connection with others
	25. Lack of peace of mind
	26. Lack of comforting rituals
Score range for Subscale 6: 0–18	27. Inability to accept realities of life
Total score range for all 27 items: 0–81	

Melancholic Behavior

Emotional processing and the ability to experience an emotion, such as sadness, are present through end-stage Alzheimer's dementia because the emotional centers of the brain are preserved [7]. Sadness, tearfulness, motor retardation, withdrawn behavior, lack of interest, and lack of motivation are common features of depression in older adults who have developed dementia [9–14].

Disagreeable Behavior

Agitation, irritability, and lack of insight are associated with depression in older adults who experience dementia [10,11,13,15,16]. Denial may be related to disagreeable behavior, which manifests itself in one of two ways: (1) an aggressive, agitated manner, or (2) a passively resistant, pessimistic manner [17,18]. Bahro and colleagues [19] reported seven case studies of older adults with Alzheimer's disease and found that avoidance, circumstantiality, cynicism, denial, detachment, displacement, irritation, normalization, sarcasm, and vagueness were used to deal with the diagnosis of Alzheimer's disease. Fisher and colleagues [20] studied cognitively impaired older adults' coping and found that behavioral disengagement was used often to cope with stressors. Older adults who experience early-stage dementia and have insight into their situation tend to maintain insight as the disease progresses even though verbal abilities decline [17].

Anxiety

Anxiety is common in individuals who have early-stage Alzheimer's disease as they consider the illness and the implications for the future [11,21]. Between 31% and 60% of older adults who experience dementia and who have depression display anxious behavior [22]. Guilt may also be present [13]. As the disease progresses and older adults are less able to communicate verbally, anxiety may be manifested by agitation or irritability. Ultimately, anxiety can exacerbate cognitive deficits [15,21]. Older adults who develop anxiety are often prescribed benzodiazepines for more than 30 days, creating cognitive deterioration, agitation, and increased risk for falls, when in reality their anxiety is a manifestation of unidentified and untreated depression [14].

Sleep Impairment

Altered sleep patterns—early morning awakening and disturbed sleep-wake patterns in particular—are common in individuals who develop dementia and are depressed [10,14,21]. Other sleep problems that may occur include difficulty falling asleep and staying asleep and sleepiness during the day [14].

Appetite Impairment

Older adults who experience dementia and are depressed often have a concomitant weight change, typically weight loss [10, 12–14]; however, weight loss or gain and decreased or increased appetite may be symptoms of depression.

Lack of Meaning in Life

Hopelessness [10,13,23], suicidal ideation [10,18,23], a lack of connection with others, loneliness, and lack of control over life may be aspects of depression in older adults. Old age is associated with various cognitive, financial, functional, physical, and social losses. An individual may make sense out of these age-related losses by finding meaning and purpose in life or by being unable to find a sense of purpose, hope, or reason for living [23].

The lifecourse perspective posits that development continues across the life span and focuses on individuals' decision-making; family and interpersonal relationships; transitions; and historical, societal, and economic contexts that influence aging [24]. For example, one older adult who has lost a spouse and is bereaved may experience impaired memory, anxiety, unresolved grief, and feelings of overwhelming panic and sorrow, whereas another older adult may adjust with relative ease [9]. Clinicians using a lifecourse perspective include family, friends, and other health care providers in their assessment to evaluate, holistically, older adults who develop dementia for depression.

Like cognitively intact older adults, individuals with Alzheimer's disease struggle to find meaning in their life and make sense out of their situation [19]. Although people who develop dementia may have difficulty communicating their feelings, a study by Waite and colleagues [6] of 72 older adults experiencing dementia revealed that 62% of individuals who had experienced a severely threatening or disturbing life event in the preceding 3 months were depressed, whereas only 28% of those who had not experienced a similar event were depressed ($P = .005$).

Recognizing suicidal ideation and behavior is essential when assessing older adults who experience dementia for depression. In industrialized countries, men who are 75 years and older have the highest suicide rates of all age groups. Factors related to suicide in older adults are feelings of anxiety, hopelessness, irritability, and worthlessness; having a serious health problem, such as dementia; experiencing a major loss; living alone; and having difficulty communicating feelings of wanting to die in a clear and direct manner [25].

INSTRUMENTATION AS AN ADJUNCT TO CLINICAL EVALUATION

Because symptoms of depression in older adults, such as decreased energy and weight, may result from disease processes or side effects of medications, correctly identifying depression in older adults can be challenging. Additionally, when older adults have dementia, they may have difficulty understanding and articulating their feelings; therefore, instruments to assess older adults for depression serve as an invaluable adjunct to health care providers' clinical judgment [14]. Many clinicians struggle with the most appropriate instrument to use to assess cognitively impaired older adults for depression. Some considerations in deciding which instrument to use to identify depression in this population include:

- Are self-rated or interviewer-rated assessment instruments preferable?
- What instruments have been designed for use in this population?
- Does the assessment instrument guide treatment?

Are Self-rated or Interviewer-rated Assessment Instruments Preferable?

Research indicates that interviewer-rated instruments are preferable to self-rated instruments in assessing older adults who have dementia for depression. Snow and colleagues [26] examined the reliability and validity of self-reported depression in older adults who have dementia and found that older adults who have dementia and depression under-reported depressive symptoms when compared with clinicians and informants. Specifically, 121 subjects from a Houston Veterans Affairs nursing home, a geropsychiatric inpatient unit, and a geropsychiatric outpatient unit were divided into four groups (37 with dementia only, 28 with depression only, 29 with depression and dementia, and 27 with neither dementia or depression). Self-reported under-identification of depressive symptoms was associated significantly with deficit awareness, the ability of an individual to accurately evaluate and report their abilities and limitations, but was not associated with severity of the cognitive impairment, physical disability, functional status, and caregiver burden. Bedard and colleagues [27] researched 1465 older adults and found that self-report instruments are invalid in individuals with a Mini-Mental State Examination Score lower than 20. The three measures of validity used were: (1) inability of individuals to respond to some questions (eg, unanswered questions on the 30-item Geriatric Depression Scale [GDS]); (2) responding positively to questions with positive wording; and (3) randomness of mood over time indicating a lack of insight into one's own feelings. Ott and Fogel [16] investigated 50 outpatients who had dementia using the self-rated GDS and the interviewer-rated Cornell Scale for Depression in Dementia and found that use of the self-rated scale with patients who experienced mild and moderate dementia underestimated the presence and degree of depression. The investigators suggest that lack of insight as dementia progresses tends to impair the ability of older adults to accurately answer self-rated questionnaires about depressive symptoms. Burke and colleagues [28] studied 142 patients using the GDS and found that it was not a valid measure for depression in older adults who had dementia and did no better than chance in identifying older adults who had mild dementia and also were depressed. These four research studies concur with psychogerontologic experts who assert that self-rated instruments may not be accurate in identifying depression in cognitively impaired older adults [2,15].

Interviewer-rated instruments are designed to ask older adults questions about their mood while providing clinicians with the opportunity to observe affect and behavior and can be used in cases of mild, moderate, and severe dementia. Observational symptoms of depression in dementia include changes in face, voice, body, and activity level. Older adults who have dementia retain the ability to express all of the basic emotions regardless of the severity of the dementia; however, the ways in which they express their emotions may change as verbal and cognitive abilities decline. To obtain the most accurate assessment, clinicians using interviewer-rated instruments may gather data from health records, inpatient or outpatient health care providers, and friends and family members [1,3,28]. Clinicians then use information from each of these sources (older adults' comments, affect, and behavior; health records; health care providers; and friends and family members) to identify patterns and inconsistencies. The assessment of depression in older adults who have dementia may require observation over a period of time to provide opportunities for behavioral comparison [29].

What Instruments Have Been Designed for Use in This Population?

Several instruments are available for assessment of depression in older adults with dementia (Table 2). Self-rated instruments are easy to administer while interviewer-rated instruments require training and take more time to administer

Table 2
Instruments to assess older adults with dementia for depression

Instrument	Author and year developed	Population	Rater
HRS-D	Hamilton, 1967	Adults of all ages (not specific to older adults)	Interviewer-rated
GDS	Brink et al, 1982	Older adults who are cognitively intact	Self-rated
CSDD	Alexopoulos et al, 1988	Older adults who have dementia	Interviewer-rated
DMAS	Sunderland et al, 1988	Older adults who have dementia	Interviewer-rated
DSA	Onega, 2004	Older adults regardless of their cognitive status	Interviewer-rated
SMI	Burton and Crossley, 2003	Older adults who have dementia	Family-rated (More of a self-rated than interviewer-rated instrument)

Abbreviations: CSDD, Cornell Scale for Depression in Dementia; DMAS, Dementia Mood Assessment Scale; DSA, Depressive Symptom Assessment for older Adults; GDS, Geriatric Depression Scale; HRS-D, Hamilton Rating Scale for Depression; SMI, Saskatchewan Mood Inventory.
   Data from Refs. [7,29,30,32,33].

but have been shown to be more accurate than self-rated instruments in this population.

Two instruments that are listed have not been designed specifically for older adults who have dementia, the Hamilton Rating Scale for Depression (HRS-D) and the GDS. Although the 17-item HRS-D is the gold standard interviewer-rated instrument for assessing adults of all ages for depression, it was not designed specifically for older adults [30,31]. The GDS is a 30-item self-rated instrument that requires either a yes or no answer to each question. The GDS does not have an item inquiring about suicidal thoughts and does not emphasize behavior or somatic symptoms [16,32].

Alexopoulos and colleagues [29] developed the Cornell Scale for Depression in Dementia (CSDD). The CSDD is a 19-item interviewer-rated instrument that uses information from interviews with a nursing staff member and the older adult. The clinician interviews the older adult's caregiver on each of the 19 items and then interviews the older adult. If there is disagreement on any of the items between the caregiver and the older adult, the clinician interviews the caregiver again and attempts to clarify the reason for the disagreement. The CSDD is scored on the basis of the clinician's judgment. Administration time is approximately 30 minutes, 20 minutes with the caregiver and 10 minutes with the older adult. Interrater reliability was $k_w = 0.67$, and internal consistency coefficient alpha was 0.84. Total CSDD scores correlated 0.83 with depressive subtypes classified according to Research Diagnostic Criteria.

The Dementia Mood Assessment Scale (DMAS) was developed based on the HRS-D, one of the oldest and most widely used scales for the measurement of depression in adults, but was designed for older adults who have dementia. The DMAS does not include subjective components, is rated on a six-point severity scale, and has 24 items with items 1 to 17 that assess for depression and items 18 to 24 that assess for severity of dementia. Four factors explained 70% of the variance: (1) depression, (2) social interaction, (3) anxiety, and (4) vegetative symptoms. Additionally, the DMAS had a correlation coefficient of 0.75 when compared with global depression ratings [33,34].

The Depressive Symptom Assessment for Older Adults (DSA) was developed in 1998 by merging the HRS-D, an interviewer-rated instrument for adults, with the DMAS, an interviewer-rated instrument for older adults who experience dementia [35–37]. The goal was to use the DSA with older adults regardless of their cognitive status. The HRS-D and the DMAS had been given to 168 community-based older adults. The 17-item version of the DMAS was used because those 17 items measure mood; the last 7 items of the DMAS were not used since they measure cognition. All 17-items of the HRS-D and all 17-items measuring mood of the DMAS were re-scaled to a consistent metric of 0 to 3. After similar items were merged to reduce redundancy, and items that were not statistically or conceptually linked to other items were dropped, 22 items were retained. The instrument was pilot-tested with 55 community-dwelling older adults; a second interviewer observed and scored interviews for 21 older adults. Interrater reliability for the total instrument was: Pearson r = 0.94, Kendall's Tau = 0.76; Subscale 1: Melancholic Behavior r = 0.92, Kendall's Tau = 0.80; Subscale 2: Disagreeable Behavior r = 0.91, Kendall's Tau = 0.80; Subscale 3: Anxiety r = 0.88, Kendall's Tau = 0.90; Subscale 4: Sleep Impairment r = 0.94, Kendall's Tau = 0.79; Subscale 5: Appetite Impairment r = 0.84, Kendall's Tau = 0.79. During interviews it became evident that the DSA was missing some important elements of depression in older adults that were not captured by other depression instruments; therefore, between 2000 and 2004 a thorough review of literature and consultation with psychogerontologic experts was done, and Subscale 6: Lack of Meaning in Life was added to the instrument.

Burton and Crossley [7] developed the Saskatchewan Mood Inventory (SMI) that was designed to be used by caregivers to identify emotional responses that the older adult who develops dementia experiences. The SMI was evaluated using 25 caregivers and was helpful in determining patterns of behavior and considering emotional reactions in their context.

Does the Assessment Instrument Guide Treatment?

Researchers often use instruments as outcome measures in evaluating nonpharmacologic interventions whereby the change in scale score is compared pre- and post-treatment [38]; however, assessment instruments can serve as guides in selecting which treatments most appropriately match the symptoms identified [14]. Instruments, such as the DSA and the SMI, are designed to enable clinicians and family members to use the assessment to guide treatment, and they hold promise for helping health care providers individualize treatment of depression in older adults who experience dementia.

ASSESSMENT OF DEPRESSION IN NURSING HOMES

Depression is a major mental health issue for nursing home residents [38]; therefore, some psychogerontologic experts propose mandatory depression screening in nursing homes to improve treatment outcomes [13]. Shah and colleagues [18] recommend required depression screening for all hospitalized older adults. Others suggest that older adults should be assessed routinely for depression as outpatients. Regardless of whether mandatory screening for depression in older adults is instituted in nursing homes, hospitals, or outpatient clinics, strategies to improve recognition of depression in older adults who have dementia are needed because identification and subsequent treatment of depression improves functional ability [26].

The Minimum Data Set Depression Rating Scale (MDSDRS), which is used in nursing homes receiving federal reimbursement, was compared with the HRS-D and the GDS in 145 nursing home residents in three Iowa nursing homes and was not found to be valid in assessing nursing home residents, 21% of whom were cognitively impaired and had depression [39]. Another study compared the 16 items under the Depression, Anxiety, and Sad Mood Indicators that are part of the mood and behavior pattern assessment of the Minimum Data Set (MDS) to the CSDD in 321 residents in three southeastern nursing homes. Fifty-three percent of the older adults had dementia; of those, 25% were identified as depressed. The MDS did not measure depressive symptoms adequately, whereas the CSDD did [15]. Cohen and colleagues [40] examined outcomes related to institution of mandatory depression screening of older adults in nursing homes who have dementia using four ethnically diverse nursing homes in New York City. Two nursing homes served as the experimental settings where mandatory depression screening was instituted (n = 519), and two served as control settings where mandatory depression screening was not done (n = 363). One of the nursing homes that served as a control was unique in that it had three consulting psychologists and three psychiatrists who spent a great deal of time with patients and provided education for staff, and most of the residents at this site were white. Results of the study showed that clinical staff can be trained to use an interviewer-rated instrument such as the CSDD. Additionally, 100% of referred individuals with dementia who were depressed were seen by a psychiatrist, which resulted in an increased use of antidepressants. Although white patients were more likely to receive antidepressants than nonwhite patients, mandatory screening increased the proportion of nonwhite individuals who received antidepressants. These three studies indicate that mandatory screening for depression in nursing homes is effective; however, the MDS does not identify depressive symptoms in older nursing home residents who have dementia adequately and should not be used to identify depression in this population. The American Geriatrics Society and American Association for Geriatric Psychiatry [41] made recommendations regarding the assessment of depression in nursing homes (Box 1):

INDIVIDUALIZED CARE FOR OLDER ADULTS WITH DEMENTIA WHO ARE DEPRESSED

Treatment for depression and depressive symptoms can improve quality of life, decrease health care costs, and improve cognitive functioning [13,21]. Some of the available treatment options are: supportive counseling to learn how to cope with deficits [13,14,20,21,25,42]; cognitive-behavioral therapy [13,20,21,25,42]; increasing social supports; establishing structured activities [13,21]; psychotherapy [14,25,38]; outdoor therapeutic recreation; bright light (10,000 lux) therapy [38]; education [14,42]; life review [14]; occupational therapy; diversional therapy; support groups [42]; referring individuals, families, and caregivers to their local chapter of the Alzheimer's Disease and Related Disorders Association for information and support services [13,14,21]; and antidepressant medications [5,13,14,21,25]. Electroconvulsive therapy is effective in treating depression in this population; however, some clinicians are concerned about adverse effects on dementia because the pathology of dementia is poorly understood [5,11,25].

Individualized care should be provided with compassion, and clinicians should determine whether nonpharmacologic or pharmacologic treatments are needed [6,14,20]. A person-centered approach for care for the older adult who has Alzheimer's disease should follow the progression outlined in Box 2 [13].

BEHAVIORAL ASSESSMENT

Affective and behavioral changes associated with Alzheimer's disease are thought to be related to the degeneration of the major brainstem aminergic

---

Box 1: Recommendations for assessing depression in nursing homes

- Screening for depression in nursing homes should be conducted 2 to 4 weeks after admission and repeated at least every 6 months.
- Depression screening instruments should be used for the identification and assessment of depressed residents and to evaluate treatment effectiveness.
- Self-report scales should be used only in cognitively intact residents, whereas interviewer-rated instruments should be used if cognitive impairment is present.
- The MDS is not adequate for the identification and treatment of depression in older adults.
- Mental health referrals should be made for suicidal ideation, psychotic depression, or depression that has not responded to treatment in 6 weeks.
- Provision of meaningful activities, volunteering, religious activities, activities that maintain past roles, and group and individual cognitive behavioral therapy may be helpful.
- Providers who are qualified and able to provide assessment and treatment in nursing homes should be reimbursed for delivering these services

---

Box 2: Care progression for a person-centered approach to Alzheimer's disease

1. Use an instrument specifically designed for this population to identify depressive symptoms or clusters of symptoms.
2. Evaluate the severity of the symptoms or clusters of symptoms.
3. Initiate nonpharmacologic and pharmacologic treatments that match the individual's symptoms and level of severity.
4. Maintain treatment while evaluating depressive symptoms and level of severity of depression.
5. Modify treatment based on symptoms and severity of symptoms.

---

nuclei that is characteristic in this disease [3]. Although this information is helpful, basic research is focused on understanding and treating the cognitive decline brought on by Alzheimer's disease; however, the behavioral sequelae of Alzheimer's disease can be disturbing to individuals, their families, and their caregivers. Clinicians need to be adept at assessing and designing interventions to address challenging behaviors [21].

When a new behavior, such as agitation, surfaces, an evaluation to rule out delirium, which is a medical emergency, should be done to be certain that the new behavior is not associated with an infection, dehydration, or medication [14,21,41,43–45]. Once delirium has been ruled out, environmental, psychosocial, and medical factors that may be exacerbating behavioral symptoms associated with dementia need to be considered. Stressors in the older adults' life should also be noted.

The prevalence of behavioral symptoms in older adults who have dementia ranges from 43% to 93% [14,45]. The Minimum Data Set is inadequate in characterizing verbal, nonverbal, and physical behavioral symptoms [41]; however, clinicians typically do not need instruments to identify dementia-related behavioral symptoms as these are easily recognizable [38]. Consequences of behavioral symptoms may include burnout or injuries to care providers, falls, isolation of the older adult, psychotropic medication administration, and use of restraints [14].

Agitation

Agitation occurs in 86% to 87% of nursing home residents who experience dementia. Specifically, 86% of older adults who have Alzheimer's disease display verbal agitation, and 55% display physical agitation [45]. Agitation is the most common behavioral challenge experienced in middle and late-stage Alzheimer's disease and often is manifested by assault, cursing, dressing and undressing, head banging, pacing, hiding, hoarding, repetitive actions, screaming, and walking aimlessly [13,21,38].

Environmental factors that increase agitation include changes in surroundings, such as moving furniture, excessive noise, or poor lighting. Stress or frustration may be associated with tasks that create a feeling of failure; therefore, examining events surrounding periods of agitation often provides insights into the causes of agitated behavior [21]. Interventions include psychotropic medication and activities that use sensory stimulation, such as music that the person enjoys and an activity, like exercise. Typically, behavior modification is not useful [38].

Perspectives for Viewing Behavioral Symptoms

Various perspectives have been developed to help clinicians view behavioral symptoms of older adults who have dementia in a therapeutic manner (Table 3). Depending on the situation, clinicians may select the perspective that they find most useful.

Rader [46] suggests adopting four roles to facilitate understanding behavioral symptoms associated with dementia and problem-solving to diminish adverse consequences of these behaviors to older adults and caregivers. The four roles are: (1) magician, (2) detective, (3) carpenter, and (4) jester. In the role of magician, the clinician sees the world from the older adult's perspective in an attempt to make sense of the behavior. As a detective, the clinician searches to identify unmet needs and evaluate the situation thoroughly to determine the cause of the behavior. When functioning as a carpenter, the nurse has a toolbox of interventions or strategies that are used to address the behavior. When dealing with behavioral symptoms of dementia, it is essential to be a jester and maintain a good sense of humor.

Treatment of Behavioral Symptoms

Whether the setting is community-based or a nursing home, strategies for care of behavioral symptoms associated with dementia should be individualized and may include kind communication, distraction, and relaxation [45]. Examples of nonpharmacologic therapy are activity therapy, environmental modifications, personalizing activities of daily living to meet individual needs [41], reminiscence [45,47], sensory therapy, and social interventions. Atypical antipsychotics are the first line of pharmacologic treatment and should be evaluated every 6 months for tapering or discontinuation. Additional medications that may be used are conventional antipsychotics, anticonvulsants, selective serotonin-reuptake inhibitors, and short- and intermediate-acting benzodiazepines [41]. In nursing homes, staff education, interdisciplinary treatment, family involvement, and mental health referrals for persistent symptoms are essential components of care [41].

To provide safe care for older adults in nursing homes who have dementia, the National Citizens' Coalition for Nursing Home Reform and the Hartford Center for Geriatric Nursing concur that staffing ratios need to be at least 4.1 hours of direct care a day. Less than 10% of nursing homes, however, meet this standard [48].

An Innovative Model of Care

Snoezelen is an individualized 24-hour program to address the behavior and mood of older adults who have developed dementia. Seventeen indicators of

Table 3
Perspectives for viewing behavioral symptoms of dementia

Perspective	Key points
ABC	• "A" stands for identifying antecedents to the behavior and determining whether they could be removed or modified. • "B" stands for evaluating the behavior—frequency, time of day, and duration. • "C" stands for determining consequences of the behavior to ascertain whether the behavior is helpful, neutral, or harmful to the individual.
Comprehensive model	• A hierarchy of causes of behavioral symptoms is considered: (1) the dementia disease process; (2) the person's underlying personality; (3) primary consequences of dementia including depression, functional impairment, delusions, and hallucinations; (4) secondary consequences of dementia including anxiety, dependence in activities of daily living, lack of meaningful activities, and spatial disorientation; and (5) behavioral symptoms of dementia associated with caregiving, social and physical environments, and medical interventions. • Consequences of dementia should be targeted for treatment.
Habilitation approach	• Goals are to promote functioning, independence, and morale. • The six domains where positive emotions are emphasized are: (1) physical environment; (2) communication; (3) functional assistance; (4) social; (5) perceptual; and (6) behavioral. • Strategies include distraction, validation of feelings, cues to promote orientation, and elimination of behavioral triggers.
NDB	• Behavioral symptoms are viewed from the older adult's perspective. • Behaviors come from a need or goal of the individual. • Environmental factors may be changed to help meet needs.
PLST	• Symptoms are divided into four groups: (1) cognitive losses; (2) affective changes; (3) planning losses; (4) and low stress threshold, which may cause behavioral symptoms. • Five stressors increase dementia-related behavior: (1) fatigue; (2) environmental, caregiver, or routine changes; (3) misleading or inappropriate stimuli; (4) demands that exceed ability; and (5) physical stressors.
Psychiatric model	• A biopsychosocial perspective is used, which includes behavioral, environmental, and pharmacologic interventions. • Medications, such as anticonvulsants, antidepressants, antipsychotics, anxiolytics, and benzodiazepines are administered depending on the individual's symptom profile.
Snoezelen (multisensory simulation)	• An individualized 24-hour program based on family history taking and stimulus preference screening demonstrates improvement in apathetic behavior, loss of decorum, rebellious behavior, aggressive behavior, and depression. • Personalized care occurs by means of caregiver training and organizational adaptations.

Abbreviations: ABC, antecedent-behaviour-consequences; NDB, need-driven dementia-compromised behaviour; PLST, Progressively lowered stress threshold.

Adapted from van Weert JC, van Dulmen AM, Spreeuwenberg PM, et al. Behavioral and mood effects of Snoezelen integrated into 24-hour dementia care. J Am Geriatr Soc 2005;53(1):24–33; and Volicer L, Hurley AC. Management of behavioral symptoms in progressive degenerative dementias. J Gerontol. Series A: Biological Sciences and Medical Sciences 2003;58A(9):837–45.

negative social psychology, such as infantilization and ignoring, and 12 indicators of positive social psychology, such as recognition and validation, serve as underpinnings of Snoezelen. This program is a person-oriented, multisensory stimulation approach that enables caregivers to incorporate lifestyle, preferences, desires, and cultural diversity into the care provided [49]. Van Weert and colleagues [49] used a quasi-experimental design to examine Snoezelen in 24-hour care in six experimental psychogeriatric wards and six control wards in Dutch nursing homes over 18 months. Residents who received Snoezelen demonstrated significantly more improvements with respect to their level of apathetic behavior, loss of decorum, rebellious behavior, aggressive behavior, and depression than the control group who received the standard care. During morning care, older adults who received Snoezelen showed more happiness and enjoyment; were in a better mood; related better to the certified nursing assistant; were more responsive to speaking; talked more frequently with normal-length sentences; and showed less inactive behavior, negativism, and reluctance than those who received the usual care. The intervention included caregiver training, implementation in daily care, stimulus preference screening of residents, writing a Snoezel care plan, and supervision meetings.

ISSUES RELATED TO PSYCHOEMOTIONAL AND BEHAVIORAL STATUS

Health service models that address the psychoemotional and behavioral needs of older adults with dementia should be instituted and evaluated. For example, one model is the use of a master's prepared mental health nurse, psychologist, or social worker to deal with mental health issues in primary care [5]. Currently, the Prevention of Suicide in Primary Care Elderly Collaborative Trial (PROSPECT) is evaluating the effectiveness of nonphysician depression care managers in primary care practices [25]. An example of a model for nursing homes is an advanced practice psychiatric nurse providing services such as staff education, psychiatric assessment and counseling, and group therapy sessions, to nursing homes [38].

Wagenaar and colleagues [50] used a Delphi technique with 10 geriatric psychiatry, geriatric psychology, and primary care medicine experts to evaluate the importance and feasibility of incorporating Agency for Health Care Policy and Research (AHCPR) guidelines for the treatment of depression in the care of nursing home residents (Table 4). Experts agreed about the importance and feasibility of two of the three assessment strategies that they were asked about; however, they did not believe that either treatment strategy that they thought was important was actually feasible. Incorporating innovations and evidenced-based care into practice settings remains an ongoing challenge.

To understand older adults' perspectives about assessment and treatment of depression, phase three of Onega's 2004 study was a 2-hour focus group of seven older adults to learn their answers to the questions in Box 3.

Themes that emerged from the discussion were that health care providers need to have a caring relationship with their older adult patients; clinicians

Table 4
Importance versus feasibility of implementing depression guidelines

Important	Feasible
Importance and feasibility matched	
Panelists thought that older adults should be assessed for suicidal ideation and attempts, anxiety, depressed mood, increase or decrease in psychomotor energy, lack of interest or pleasure, lack of reactivity to pleasant stimuli, early morning awakening, weight change, and anhedonia.	Panelists believed that it was feasible to assess older adults for suicidal ideation and attempts, anxiety, comorbid medical illnesses, psychotic symptoms, and dementia symptoms. Additionally, most of them thought symptoms of depressed mood, psychomotor energy changes, lack of interest and reactivity, diurnal mood variation, and weight change were feasible to obtain.
Importance and feasibility did NOT match	
Experts thought that the GDS was important to use for the diagnosis of depression in older adults. They did not believe that the MDS, the CSDD, or the CES-D Scale were important for diagnostic purposes.	Ninety percent believed that obtaining the MDS was feasible, whereas only 10% rated the GDS, CSDD, or CES-D as feasible to obtain in the nursing home.
Importance and feasibility matched	
Laboratory assessment varied in importance with complete blood count, electrolytes, B_{12} level, and thyroid stimulating hormone being selected as most important.	All panelists believed that obtaining laboratory values was feasible.
Importance and feasibility did NOT match	
All panelists believed that psychotherapy and antidepressants were important for treating older adults who had depression in nursing homes.	Although all of the panelists believed that a combination of psychotherapy and antidepressants were important, none of the experts believed that it was feasible to obtain combination therapy. Ten percent of the group believed that psychotherapy was feasible; 80% believed that antidepressant medication without psychotherapy was feasible.
Importance and feasibility did NOT match	
ECT was considered an important treatment option.	Eighty percent believed that it was not feasible to arrange ECT for nursing home residents.

Abbreviations: CES-D, Center for Epidemiologic Studies Depression; ECT, electrocovulsive therapy.
   Adapted from Wagenaar D, Colenda CC, Kreft M, et al. Treating depression in nursing homes: practice guidelines in the real world. J Am Osteopath Assoc 2003;103(10):465–69,498–99.

should monitor older adults' symptoms and evaluate the effectiveness of treatment; health care providers, patients, and families need to be educated about how to recognize and treat depression; nurses should assist older adults to find ways of engaging and connecting with other people; and health care encounters with older adults should not be rushed. One participant suggested that clinicians may find it helpful to look through an older adult's photo album

Box 3: Questions asked older adults about assessment and treatment of depression in Onega's 2004 study

1. What are health care providers currently doing to identify depression in their older adult patients?

2. What are some of the reasons that health care providers may not identify depression in their older adult patients who are depressed?

3. What do you think that health care providers could do to improve their ability to identify older adults who are depressed?

4. What strategies are most helpful for health care providers to use in treating depression in their older adult patients?

5. What strategies are least helpful for health care providers to use in treating depression in their older adult patients?

6. How do Medicare and other types of insurance influence the treatment of depression in older adults?

7. What other comments or thoughts about depression in older adults would you like to share?

with him/her because it is difficult for patients to find words to express their feelings. He pulled out a small photo album and showed it to the group. Throughout the album there were pictures of him with his wife hiking in the mountains together. At the time of the study his wife had dementia and was living in a dementia care unit, and he lived independently but used a walker. By looking through the photo album it was clear that hiking and being in nature with his wife had been important to him. He suggested that health care providers use this strategy to identify profound losses and help individuals find ways of mitigating some of their losses.

SUMMARY

Many older adults who have dementia also have depression and behavioral symptoms that interfere with their functioning, decrease their quality of life, and add to their health care costs. Recognizing depressive symptoms in older adults who experience dementia is challenging; therefore, clinicians may find it helpful to use an interviewer-rated instrument as an adjunct to their clinical judgment. Various perspectives have been developed to help clinicians view behavioral symptoms of older adults who have dementia in a therapeutic manner. Compassionate, individualized care for depression and behavioral symptoms should be provided that addresses the presenting symptoms.

Acknowledgments
    1. Part of this work was funded by a Waldron Research Award for the study Content Validation of the Depressive Symptom Assessment for Older Adults
    2. Special thanks to Judy Murray, MSW, for her assistance with data analysis.

References

[1] Alexopoulos GS. Depression and other mood disorders. Clinical Geriatrics 2000;8(11): 69–72, 75–8, 81–2.

[2] Alexopoulos GS, Katz IR, Reynolds CF, et al. Pharmacotherapy of depression in older patients: a summary of the expert consensus guidelines. J Psychiatr Pract 2001;7(6): 361–76.

[3] Zubenko GS, Zubenko WN, McPherson S, et al. A collaborative study of the emergence and clinical features of the major depressive syndrome of Alzheimer's disease. Am J Psychiatry 2003;160(5):857–66.

[4] Alexopoulos GS, Katz IR, Reynolds CF, et al. Depression in older adults. J Psychiatr Pract 2001;7(6):441–6.

[5] Reynolds CF, Alexopoulos GS, Katz IR, et al. Chronic depression in the elderly: approaches for prevention. Drugs Aging 2001;18(7):507–14.

[6] Waite A, Bebbington P, Skelton-Robinson M, et al. Life events, depression and social support in dementia. Br J Clin Psychol 2004;43(3):313–24.

[7] Burton C, Crossley M. Examining the utility of the Saskatchewan Mood Inventory for individuals with memory loss. Can J Aging 2003;22(3):297–309.

[8] Lynn MR. Determination and quantification of content validity. Nurs Res 1986;35(6): 382–6.

[9] Khin NA, Sunderland T. Bereavement in older adults: biological, functional and psychological consequences. Psychiatric Times 2000;17(1):47–8.

[10] McAndrew C, Vandivort M. The six principles of excellent clinical care for dementia: nurse practitioners and physicians working together. Nurse Pract Forum 2001;12(1):12–22.

[11] O'Brien J. Behavioral symptoms in vascular cognitive impairment and vascular dementia. Int Psychogeriatr 2003;15(Suppl 1):133–8.

[12] Onalaja D, Sikabofori T, Jainer AK. Differentiating depression from dementia in the elderly. Geriatric Medicine 2004;34(6):67–71.

[13] Rabheru K. Depression in dementia: diagnosis and treatment. Psychiatric Times 2004;21(13) Special Report: Comorbidities:33–4, 38–9.

[14] Voyer P, Martin LS. Improving geriatric mental health nursing care: making a case for going beyond psychotropic medications. Int J Ment Health Nurs 2003;12(1):11–21.

[15] Hendrix CC, Sakauye KM, Karabatsos G, et al. The use of the Minimum Data Set to identify depression in the elderly. J Am Med Dir Assoc 2003;4(6):308–12.

[16] Ott BR, Fogel BS. Measurement of depression in dementia: self vs clinician rating. Int J Geriatr Psychiatry 1992;7(12):899–904.

[17] Arkin SM, Mahendra N. Geriatric Depression Scale as dementia insight indicator: three case examples. Clin Gerontol 2003;26(3/4):171–5.

[18] Shah A, Dighe-Deo D, Chapman C, et al. Suicidal ideation amongst acutely medically ill and continuing care geriatric inpatients. Aging Ment Health 1998;2(4):300–5.

[19] Bahro M, Silber E, Sunderland T. How do patients with Alzheimer's disease cope with their illness? A clinical experience report. J Am Geriatr Soc 1995;43(1):41–6.

[20] Fisher BM, Segal DL, Coolidge FL. Assessment of coping in cognitively impaired older adults: a preliminary study. Clin Gerentol 2003;26(3/4):3–12.

[21] Lawlor BA, Sunderland T. Alzheimer's disease: a strategy for coping with behavioral changes. Consultant 1994;34(1):43–6.

[22] Gardner ME, Malone DC, Sey M, et al. Mirtazapine is associated with less anxiolytic use among elderly depressed patients in long-term care facilities. J Am Med Dir Assoc 2004;5(2):101–6.

[23] Ron P. Depression, hopelessness, and suicidal ideation among the elderly: a comparison between men and women living in nursing homes and in the community. J Gerontol Soc Work 2004;43(2/3):97–116.

[24] Turner MJ, Killian TS, Cain R. Life course transitions and depressive symptoms among women in midlife. Int J Aging Hum Dev 2004;58(4):241–65.

[25] Szanto K, Gildengers A, Mulsant BH, et al. Identification of suicidal ideation and prevention of suicidal behaviour in the elderly. Drugs Aging 2002;19(1):11–24.

[26] Snow AL, Kunik ME, Molinari VA, et al. Accuracy of self-reported depression in persons with dementia. J Am Geriatr Soc 2005;53(3):389–96.

[27] Bedard M, Molloy DW, Squire L, et al. Validity of self-reports in dementia research: the Geriatric Depression Scale. Clin Gerontol 2003;26(3/4):155–63.

[28] Burke WJ, Houston MJ, Boust SJ, et al. Use of the Geriatric Depression Scale in dementia of the Alzheimer's type. J Am Geriatr Soc 1989;37(9):856–60.

[29] Alexopoulos GS, Abrams RC, Young RC, et al. Cornell Scale for Depression in Dementia. Biol Psychiatry 1988;23:271–84.

[30] Hamilton M. Development of a rating scale for primary depressive illness. Br J Soc Clin Psychol 1967;6(4):278–96.

[31] Onega LL, Abraham IL. Factor structure of the Hamilton Rating Scale for Depression in a cohort of community-dwelling elderly. Int J Geriatr Psychiatry 1997;12(7):760–4.

[32] Brink TL, Yesavage JA, Lum O, et al. Screening tests for geriatric depression. Clin Gerontol 1982;1(1):37–43.

[33] Sunderland T, Alterman IS, Yount D, et al. A new scale for the assessment of depressed mood in demented patients. Am J Psychiatry 1988;145(8):955–9.

[34] Sunderland T, Minichiello M. Dementia Mood Assessment Scale. Int Psychogeriatr 1996;8(Suppl 3):329–31.

[35] Onega LL, Abraham IL, Stewart B, et al. Differentiated assessment of depressive symptoms in community-dwelling elders: why, what, how, when, who? Paper presented at the meeting of the 15th Annual Oregon Rural Health Conference. Sunriver, October 17, 1998.

[36] Onega LL, Stewart BJ, Fields J. Understanding Presentations of Depression in Older Adults. Paper presented at the meeting of the Gerontological Society of America. Boston, November 22, 2002.

[37] Onega LL, Stewart B, Fields J. Presentations of depression in older adults. Poster session presented at the annual meeting of the International Psychogerontological Association. Chicago, August 19, 2003.

[38] Snowden M, Sato K, Roy-Byrne P. Assessment and treatment of nursing home residents with depression or behavioral symptoms associated with dementia: a review of the literature. J Am Geriatr Soc 2003;51(9):1305–17.

[39] Snowden M. The minimum data set depression rating scale (MDSDRS) lacks reliability for identifying depression among older adults living in nursing homes. Evid Based Ment Health 2004;7(1):7.

[40] Cohen CI, Hyland K, Kimhy D. The utility of mandatory depression screening of dementia patients in nursing homes. Am J Psychiatry 2003;160(11):2012–7.

[41] American Geriatrics Society/American Association for Geriatric Psychiatry. Consensus statement on improving the quality of mental health care in US nursing homes: management of depression and behavioral symptoms associated with dementia. J Am Geriatr Soc 2003;51(9):1287–98.

[42] Brodaty H, Lee-Fay L. Making memories: pilot evaluation of a new program for people with dementia and their caregivers. Australas J Ageing 2004;23(3):144–6.

[43] Amella EJ. Presentation of illness in older adults: if you think you know what you're looking for, think again. Am J Nurs 2004;104(10):40–52.

[44] Haymore J. A neuron in a haystack: advanced neurologic assessment. AACN Clinical Issues. Advanced Practice in Acute and Critical Care 2004;15(4):568–81.

[45] Volicer L, Hurley AC. Management of behavioral symptoms in progressive degenerative dementias. J Gerontol A Biol Sci Med Sci 2003;58A(9):837–45.

[46] Rader J. The problem-solving process. In: Individualized dementia care: creativecompassionate approaches. New York: Springer Publishing Company; 1995. p. 19–26.

[47] Moss SE, Polignano E, White CL, et al. Reminiscence group activities and discourse interaction in Alzheimer's disease. J Gerontol Nurs 2002;28(8):36–44.

[48] Lenhoff DR. The American Geriatrics Society/American Association for Geriatric Psychiatry mental health in nursing homes consensus statement. Recommendations for policies in support of quality mental health care in US nursing homes and the consensus statement on improving the quality of mental health care in US nursing homes: management of depression and behavioral symptoms associated with dementia. J Am Geriatr Soc 2003;51(9):1324.

[49] van Weert JCM, van Dulmen AM, Spreeuwenberg PM, et al. Behavioral and mood effects of Snoezelen integrated into 24-hour dementia care. J Am Geriatr Soc 2005;53(1):24–33.

[50] Wagenaar D, Colenda CC, Kreft M, et al. Treating depression in nursing homes: practice guidelines in the real world. J Am Osteopath Assoc 2003;103(10):465–9, 498–9.

ELSEVIER
SAUNDERS

Nurs Clin N Am 41 (2006) 43–55

NURSING CLINICS
OF NORTH AMERICA

Abuse and Neglect in Older Adults with Alzheimer's Disease

Carla VandeWeerd, PhD[a],*, Gregory J. Paveza, MSW, PhD[b],
Terry Fulmer, PhD, RN, FAAN[c]

[a]The James and Jennifer Harrell Center for the Study of Family Violence,
Department of Community and Family Health, College of Public Health,
University of South Florida, 13301 Bruce B Downs Boulevard, MDC 56,
Tampa, FL 33620, USA
[b]Division of Arts and Sciences, University of South Florida, Lakeland,
3433 Winter Lake Road, Lakeland, FL 33803, USA
[c]Division of Nursing, New York University, 246 Greene Street, New York,
NY 10003-6677, USA

Elder mistreatment (EM) is a serious issue that effects the lives of thousands of older adults and results in emotional difficulties, such as depression [1,2] feelings of inadequacy, self-loathing [3,4], and lowered self-esteem [3,4,5,6,7]. EM has been shown to result in family distress, impaired life functioning [2], and difficulties with cognition [5] and is linked to health problems, such as immunologic dysfunction [1,2,5,7,8], and increased mortality [9]. As the population ages, and with it the numbers of persons afflicted by diseases such as Alzheimer's disease (AD), understanding and recognizing elder mistreatment becomes an important factor in maintaining quality of life for older adults.

ELDER MISTREATMENT

EM, as defined by the National Research Council, refers to (a) intentional actions that cause harm or create a serious risk for harm (whether or not harm is intended) to a vulnerable elder by a caregiver or other person who stands in a trust relationship to an elder or (b) failures by a caregiver to satisfy the elders basic needs or to protect the elder from harm. Although there is much differentiation in state laws and research as to the exact definition of what constitutes EM, in general, five categories are distinguished [10,11,12,13,14]: (1) physical abuse or aggression, (2) sexual abuse, (3) psychologic mistreatment or chronic verbal aggression, (4) financial or material mistreatment, and (5) neglect, distinguished by perpetrator (ie, caregiver or self).

*Corresponding author. E-mail address: cvandewe@hsc.usf.edu (C. VandeWeerd).

0029-6465/06/$ – see front matter
doi:10.1016/j.cnur.2005.09.004

Regardless of varying definitional specifics, there is consensus among clinicians and researchers that EM seriously effects the lives of thousands of older adults. The most commonly cited population-based study of older adults [15] found an overall prevalence of EM to be 32 elderly persons per 1000 for an annual prevalence of 700,000 to 1.2 million cases of elder mistreatment in the United States. The recently completed National Elder Abuse Incidence Study also examined overall incidence of EM and found that approximately 551,000 persons were identified as abused or neglected in 1996, and they acknowledge that this number may be as high as 800,000. Most cases of abuse and neglect still are under-reported.

THE VULNERABILITY OF PERSONS WITH ALZHEIMER'S DISEASE

Alzheimer's disease (AD) is the most common dementing disorder in Western society [16]. As many as 10% of persons over the age of 65 may be suffering at least early stages of the disease, and as many as 30% of persons over the age of 80 may be affected and the problem is growing. By the year 2040 it is estimated that this number grow to 13 million [17,18].

AD progresses slowly, usually lasting between 5 and 15 or more years [19a]. It often starts with difficulty in functions of the mind and ends with complete loss of ability to function physically, including the loss of ability to complete most activities of daily living unassisted. AD comes with component problems in cognition that span memory, language, attention, perception, and motor skills. It includes such things as loss of attention [19a,20], loss of communication skills [21], and loss of perceptual skills, which can hinder driving, reading, and dressing [22]. AD also often includes depression, agitation, suspiciousness, delusions, and hallucinations [16].

Caring for a loved one with a cognitive impairment increases a caregivers risk for engaging in abusive behaviors [23–35]. The recently completed Aggression and Violence in Community Based Alzheimer's Disease Families study examined aggression and violence in community-residing persons with AD in the state of Florida and found that 60.1% of caregivers had been verbally abusive with the person they were providing care for and 17.2% had been violent. In light of the etiology of cognitive disease this is not surprising. As a result of the changes that stem from the disease, and their ripple effects on caregivers, traditional theories of EM support the idea that this population is at increased risk for mistreatment at the hands of their care providers.

RISK FACTORS FOR ELDER MISTREATMENT

Theories such as poor social learning, pathology of the perpetrator, internal or external stress, social isolation, disability or impairment, internal family dynamics, and inadequate exchange have been suggested in the literature in an effort to lend insight as to why abuse and neglect of older adults may occur [13,23,36–39]. These theories identify possible risk factors for EM and postulate that abuse may stem from several areas in which AD families may have an increased likelihood of being vulnerable.

Of the theories listed above, social learning theory and the theory of abuser pathology add least to the understanding of why Alzheimer's family caregivers are at increased risk for engaging in elder mistreatment. These theories postulate that mistreatment is learned, passed on from a parent to a child who then victimizes them in old age or alternatively that abusers have personality traits or characteristics that cause them to be abusive. While it is likely some elder mistreatment in persons with AD may be domestic violence grown old, there is no reason to suspect at present that persons with AD are more likely to have engaged in domestic violence than persons living in the general population [19b].

Limited evidence does exist in support of the idea that increased risk for mistreatment may be related to abuser pathology in the caregivers of dementia patients. Substance abuse by caretakers, for example, has been linked to EM in several studies [15,40–47] and a growing body of literature exists to support the idea that caregivers of AD patients may experience higher levels of burden [48,49] and may, as a result, be prone to poor coping mechanisms, such as substance abuse. Some researchers have found that the long term effects of care required by AD patients can result in the clinical manifestation of Post Traumatic Stress Disorder (PTSD) or other psychopathology in its care providers [50].

According to stress theory, caregivers may be at an increased likelihood for engaging in EM as a result of external or internal stress, which tend to be high in AD caregivers [48,49]. External stresses shown to be related to EM include being financially dependent [51], emotionally dependent [13,43,45], or housing dependent [51] on care receivers, or experiencing personal stressors, such as marital discord or financial difficulties [47]. Severe financial strain resulting from the inordinate cost of caring for a person with AD is not uncommon [16].

Internal stressors, such as burden of care [25], depression [15,23,26, 39,42,52–56], and other caregiver emotional problems [15,23,42,47] also are related to increased risk for EM. The enormous personal and time commitment required to provide care for someone with a disease course that ends with the patient needing assistance in all areas of daily living results in higher levels of internal stress, depression, and burden in AD family caregivers than those found in the general population. This stress and burden contributes significantly to an increased risk for EM [19b,57,58].

Caregiver [39,43,57,58] and patient isolation lead to an increased susceptibility to EM [59], and persons with AD and their caregivers are likely to be socially isolated. This theory postulates that social supports function as an important moderator to life stress and pathology, as a result those without social support are more likely to abuse. For care providers, social isolation may stem from the enormous amount of time care-providing requires [49], resulting in a restriction of normal activities.

Patients' isolation often stems from a result of their inability to negotiate their surroundings, communicate, or to keep "troublesome" public behaviors in check [19b,21,22]. Patients may choose to isolate themselves as a way of hiding their cognitive impairment [19b,22] and may choose to hide their abuse rather than report it for fear of the consequences [4,5,60,61]. For many persons with cognitive impairment, institutionalization represents the removal of the last of their independence, a final loss of self, and many would rather stay in an abusive situation than be institutionalized. As a result, EM may go unnoticed and untreated in this subpopulation.

Caregivers of persons with AD are also at increased risk for engaging in EM because they are providing care for someone with increased overall vulnerability. The vulnerability hypothesis, an offshoot of those listed above, supports the idea that some elders may be abused by virtue of characteristics that increase their dependence on others and so increase the stress of others caused by the burden of that strain. The fact that persons with AD are, or become, dependent on their caregivers for assistance has already been highlighted. These persons are further made vulnerable by a society that fails to recognize EM and that blames elders "inadequacy" or "incompetence" for abuse with ageist attitudes that prevent them from coming forward [3,5]. Further, it states that vulnerability is exacerbated by a decrease in their ability or willingness to guard against or escape from abuse [23]. Persons who experienced increased physical vulnerability, such as that brought on by AD, are further inhibited because they may not have good communication or physical skills. As a result of their impairment, they may not be able to make a report or to defend themselves.

Relationship between caregiver and care recipient has been identified in the literature as a significant predictor of EM [10,15,28,32,36,39,42,62]. Exchange theory holds that interaction between individuals is guided by its rewards and costs. In cases where the relationship is good, risk for EM is decreased significantly; in cases where the relationship is poor, and the laws of reciprocity and distributive justice are violated, such as in the case of AD patients, risk goes up. Persons with AD are disadvantaged because they often have less to "give" others as a result of the physical and cognitive declines associated with their disease.

During the period of the end-stages of dementia, persons with this disease especially are at risk for EM because they may be prevented, physically or cognitively, from engaging in traditional "giving" activities, such as child-care or assistance with housework while a care provider is otherwise occupied.

RECIPROCAL VIOLENCE

Although it is likely some EM in persons with AD may be domestic violence grown old, recent research has begun to show that EM may be a dyadic rather than a one-way street, with violence by AD caregivers as a prime example.

Research has shown that mistreatment on the part of caregivers often may be the result of violence inflicted upon them by the patient [25,28, 30,32,34,35,48,63]. Caregivers who have been physically or verbally abused by the patients they are providing care for, eventually succumb to using these behaviors themselves. As they are not recognized by their loved ones, called names, threatened, or are hit or bit in the course of providing care, they may engage in reciprocal mistreatment. The Aggression and Violence in Community Based Alzheimer's disease study found that 74.2% of patients had been verbally abusive to their caregiver, and 73.9% had been physically violent. Caregivers had rates of 60.1% for verbal abuse and 17.2% for violence. Before the onset of symptoms, however, these rates were much closer to the population norms. Verbal aggression was reported by only 9.6% of caregivers and 11% of patients, and violence was reported by only 2.6% of caregivers and 3.1% of patients indicating that in many of these persons mistreatment is a consequence of the disease process rather than domestic violence grown old. Although this in no way excuses these behaviors, it does lend credibility to the idea that in some cases, services rather than punishment are warranted.

ASSESSING ELDER MISTREATMENT AND NEGLECT

The American Medical Association recommends that physicians routinely observe for indicators of abuse and neglect, and inquire about EM, just as they screen for other conditions, such as cancer [64]. Any service provider coming into contact with older adults should do the same. Questions should be posed in a nonthreatening manner, and general questions, such as "who cooks for you?" or "do you get help when you need it?" should be asked and may pave the way for targeted inquiries, such as "does your daughter ever hit you when you disagree?" or "do you have to wait a long time to get food or medication?" [65]. Subjective complaints of abuse and neglect made at any time should be taken seriously and investigated immediately.

Persons who have AD may be unwilling (for fear of reprisal or institutionalization) or unable as a result of their disease condition to verbalize that abuse or neglect is going on, and providers should be aware of signs and symptoms that may signal that abuse or neglect may be occurring. Changes in financial status, such as an inability to pay bills, pay for required medications, or purchase appropriate clothing, when this has not be a problem previously may be indicative of financial abuse. Frequent visits to the emergency department, unexplained injuries or injuries inconsistent with given explanation, missed follow-up appointments, delays in receiving medical care, and malnutrition, may be indicators of physical abuse or neglect. Psychologic mistreatment may manifest itself in changes in appearance, depression, decreased self-esteem, and social withdrawal.

Several instruments exist to assist in making a diagnosis of EM. The Indicators of Abuse Screen (IOA) [66], The Hwalek-Sengstock Elder Abuse Screening Test Revised (H-S/EAST) [67], the Conflict Tactic Scale (CTS) [68], and the Elder Abuse Assessment Inventory (EAI) [69] all have been used to assess for abuse and neglect in the general population. Several of these instruments rely upon older adults responses to questions, which make them less useful as AD progresses and lucid cognition on the part of the older adult becomes more difficult. The EAI, however, heavily relies on clinical observation and judgment in its general assessment, neglect assessment, usual lifestyle and

General Assessment		Very Good	Good	Poor	Very Poor	Unable to Assess
1.	Clothing	1	2	3	4	9999
2.	Hygiene	1	2	3	4	9999
3.	Nutrition	1	2	3	4	9999
4.	Skin Integrity	1	2	3	4	9999

Neglect Assessment		No Evidence	Probably No Evidence	Probably Evidence	Evidence	Unable to Assess
5.	Bruising	1	2	3	4	9999
6.	Contractures	1	2	3	4	9999
7.	Decubiti	1	2	3	4	9999
8.	Dehydration	1	2	3	4	9999
9.	Diarrhea	1	2	3	4	9999
10.	Impaction	1	2	3	4	9999
11.	Lacerations	1	2	3	4	9999
12.	Malnutrition	1	2	3	4	9999
13.	Urine burns/excoriations	1	2	3	4	9999

Usual Lifestyle		Totally Independent	Mostly Independent	Mostly Dependent	Totally Dependent	Unable to Assess
14.	Administration of meds	1	2	3	4	9999
15.	Ambulation	1	2	3	4	9999
16.	Continence	1	2	3	4	9999
17.	Feedings	1	2	3	4	9999
18.	Maintenance of hygiene	1	2	3	4	9999
19.	Management of finances	1	2	3	4	9999
20.	Family support	1	2	3	4	9999

Social Assessment		Very Good Quality	Good Quality	Poor Quality	Very Poor Quality	Unable to Assess
21.	Financial situation	1	2	3	4	9999
22.	Interaction with family	1	2	3	4	9999
23.	Interaction with friends	1	2	3	4	9999
24.	Interaction with nursing home personnel	1	2	3	4	9999
25.	Living arrangement	1	2	3	4	9999
26.	Observed relationship with care provider	1	2	3	4	9999
27.	Participation in daily social activities	1	2	3	4	9999
28.	Support systems	1	2	3	4	9999
29.	Ability to express needs	1	2	3	4	9999

Fig. 1. Elder Abuse Assessment Inventory (EAI). *Adapted from* Fulmer T, Street S, Carr K. Abuse of the elderly: screening and detection. J Emer Nurs 1984;10(3):131–40.

Medical Assessment	No Evidence	Probably No Evidence	Probably Evidence	Evidence	Unable to Assess
30. Duplication of similar medications (e.g., multiple laxatives, sedatives)	1	2	3	4	9999
31. Unusual doses of medication	1	2	3	4	9999
32. Alcohol/substance abuse	1	2	3	4	9999
33. Greater than 15% dehydration	1	2	3	4	9999
34. Bruises and/or trauma beyond what is compatible with alleged trauma	1	2	3	4	9999
35. Failure to respond to warning of obvious disease	1	2	3	4	9999
36. Repetitive admissions due to probable failure of health care surveillance	1	2	3	4	9999

Emotional / Psychological Neglect	No Evidence	Probably No Evidence	Probably Evidence	Evidence	Unable to Assess
37. Elder states being left alone for long periods of time	1	2	3	4	9999
38. Elder states being ignored or given the "silent treatment"	1	2	3	4	9999
39. Elder states failure to receive companionship, news, changes in routine, information	1	2	3	4	9999
40. Subjective complaint of neglect	1	2	3	4	9999

Summary Assessments	No Evidence	Probably No Evidence	Probably Evidence	Evidence	Unable to Assess
41. Evidence of neglect	1	2	3	4	9999
42. Evidence of physical abuse	1	2	3	4	9999
43. Evidence of psychological abuse	1	2	3	4	9999
44. Evidence of financial abuse	1	2	3	4	9999

Disposition	Yes	No
45. Referral to social service	1	0
46. Referral to other If yes, please specify _____	1	0

Fig. 1 (continued)

medical assessments, and would serve as a helpful tool in assessing for possible physical abuse or neglect in persons across the spectrum of AD (Fig. 1). For most cases where abuse or neglect is suspected, and especially for those in mid- to end stage AD, a multi-disciplinary team assessment would be the best approach in the recognition and prevention of elder mistreatment.

Interactions with persons with AD, also often provide for interaction with their caregiver. Caregivers may be experiencing abuse at the hand of their loved one with AD or may be neglecting themselves to provide care. As a result, they too should be routinely assessed for abuse and neglect during any interaction and referred to services or intervention as appropriate.

PREVENTION AND TREATMENT

It has been suggested in the literature that unrecognized needs of persons with dementia, and the subsequent failure to meet those needs often results in a cycle of agitation and altered behaviors that can precipitate conflictual and often violent interactions between the care provider and care recipient leading to abuse [34,35,70]. They suggest that abusive situations develop in part, because the burdens of providing care, the task oriented nature of providing care, and the lack of awareness of specific intervention and communication strategies which honor the individual person and address their specific needs within the context of dementia. By creatively using and exploring differing forms of verbal and non-verbal communication, knowing their life history, preferences, and through the use of behavioral modification techniques, care providers can learn to communicate and interpret signals and behaviors from the individual with dementia, and reduce the level of conflict. Excellent guides on techniques for doing these things with persons with dementia are available [20–22]. They include suggestions for better communication, such as reducing background noise while talking and the importance of tone of voice. They also include sections on easy activities for redirecting attention, such as blowing up a balloon and playing with it. More significantly, these manuals highlight the importance of re-framing the experience, focusing on the positives of today's capabilities, being the memory keeper, and the importance of patient dignity.

To reduce stress, social isolation, and depression, pharmacologic treatment, supportive psychotherapy, education groups, and services that decrease the hours per day spent providing care (respite) may also represent effective preventative solutions [71]. Although the Alzheimer Disease Management guidelines emphasize the importance of caregiver support and nonpharmacologic intervention as necessary compliments to any pharmacologic intervention [72], a recent study of health professionals indicated that only about one third of health care professionals routinely provided support group or respite referral, telephone follow up, or behavioral coaching [73].

Additional avenues for prevention lie in education of health professionals around the importance of recognizing abuse and neglect and its risk factors. A recent study found that nearly one third of health professionals did not routinely screen for depression or routinely perform cognitive screening [73].

Pharmacologic interventions, such as antipsychotic and anxiolytic drugs are also helpful for reducing agitation and aggressive behaviors in persons who have AD [72] and may reduce the likelihood of reciprocal violence.

BARRIERS

Barriers to detecting and intervening in cases of EM revolve around issues of inconsistent and inconclusive data, lack of awareness of health professionals, and broader societal attitudes.

To date, little research as specifically focused on EM in persons who have AD. Although insight has resulted from other research that has posited several theories and advanced the understanding of issues of EM, it has not been without flaws. Researchers have pointed out that data collected on the basis of Adult Protective Service status may yield biased samples as a result of selection bias, as only those cases identified as problematic are brought to the attention of the researcher [74,75]. Reaching the oldest old and persons who experience health difficulties, has also been cited in the literature as problematic for EM research [6,76] as has the necessity to rely on secondary reporters [14] and on cross-sectional designs [10,38]. Concern for under reporting of EM as a result of subject bias toward socially desirable response has also been noted [77]. In addition, many studies focus only on victim characteristics despite the fact that abuser characteristics may be equally or more salient [10,46,67,75,76].

Lack of awareness on the part of health professionals also impedes effective recognition and treatment. The Institute of Medicine panel on the Training of Health Professionals found that less than 5% of time in schools of social work and 3% of time in schools of nursing is dedicated to education around issues of EM [78].

An unwillingness on the part of older adults and caregivers to talk about EM is also a barrier. Older adults may stay silent for fear of reprisal or for fear of being institutionalized as many see occasional neglect of mistreatment at home as being better than institutionalization. Caregivers, being abused by the person they are providing care for may also feel unwilling to come forward for fear that their loved one will be removed from the home.

SUMMARY

As the number of older adults who have AD grows, clinicians and service providers should learn to recognize it and to offer appropriate intervention. Where abuse and neglect are intentional, punitive measures are likely in order but where mistreatment stems from depression, stress, burnout, or reciprocal violence services rather than punishment are warranted.

References
[1] Light E, Lebowitz B. Alzheimer's disease treatment and family stress: directions for research. Rockville (MD): National Institute of Mental Health; 1994.
[2] Zarit S, Todd P, Zarit J. Subjective burden of husbands and wives as caregivers. A longitudinal study. Gerontologist 1986;26:260–6.

[3] Metge J. In and out of touch: Whakamaa in cross cultural perspective. Wellington (NZ): Victoria University Press; 1986.

[4] Lewis M. Shame: the exposed self. New York: The Free Press; 1992.

[5] Barer BM. The secret shame of the very old: "I've never told this to anyone else." J Ment Health Aging 1997;3(3):365–75.

[6] Comijs HC, Pot AM, Smit JH, et al. Elder abuse in the community: prevalence and consequences. J Am Geriatr Soc 1998;46(7):885–8.

[7] Saverman B. Formal careers in healthcare and social services witnessing the abuse of the elderly in their homes. Umeå, Sweden: Umeå University; 1994.

[8] George L, Gywther L. Caregiver well-being—a multidimensional examination of family caregivers of demented adults. Gerontologist 1986;26:253–9.

[9] Lachs MS, Williams CS, O'Brien S, et al. The mortality of elder mistreatment. JAMA 1998;280(5):428–32.

[10] Comijs HC, Jonker C, van Tilburg W, et al. Hostility and coping capacity as risk factors of elder mistreatment. Soc Psychiatry Psychiatr Epidemiol 1999;34(1):48–52.

[11] Lachs MS, Williams C, O'Brien S, et al. Older adults: an 11-year longitudinal study of adult protective service use. Arch Intern Med 1996;156:449–54.

[12] National Research Council. Elder mistreatment; abuse, neglect, and exploitation in an aging America. Panel to review risk and prevalence of elder abuse and neglect. In: Bonnie RJ, Wallace RB, editors. Washington, DC: The National Academic Press; 2003.

[13] Pillemer DA, Finkelhor D. Causes of elder abuse: caregiver stress versus problem relatives. Am J Orthopsychiatry 1989;59(2):179–87.

[14] Poertner J. Estimation the incidence of abused older persons. J Gerontol Soc Work 1986;9(3):3–15.

[15] Pillemer K, Finkelhor D. The prevalence of elder abuse: a random sample survey. Gerontologist 1988;28:51–7.

[16] Blazer D. Emotional problems in later life: intervention strategies for professional caregivers (2nd ed.). New York (NY): Springer Publishing Co.; 1998.

[17] Ewbank D. Alzheimer's disease as a cause of death in the US: estimates and projections. Population Aging Research Center, University of Pennsylvania, Working Paper Series No. 95–02.1995.

[18] Herbert LE, Scherr PA, Bienias JL. Alzheimer's disease in the US population: prevalence estimates using the 2000 census. Archives of Neuorology 2003;60:1119–22.

[19a] Cohen D, Eisdorfer C. The loss of self: a family resource for the care of Alzheimer's disease and related disorders. New York: W.W. Norton & Company; 1986.

[19b] Cohen D, Eisdorfer C. Depression in family members caring for a relative with Alzheimer's disease. J Am Geriatr Soc 1986;36:855–89.

[20] Bridges BJ. Therapeutic caregiving: a practical guide for caregivers of persons with Alzheimer's and other dementia causing diseases. Mill Creek (WA): BJB Publishing; 1995.

[21] Feil N. The validation breakthrough: simple techniques for communicating with people with "Alzheimer's-type dementia." Baltimore (MD): Health Professions Press; 1993.

[22] Bell V, Troxell D. The best friends approach to Alzheimer's care. Baltimore (MD): Health Professions Press; 1997.

[23] Anetzberger GJ. The etiology of elder abuse by adult offspring. Chicago: Springfield Publishing; 1987.

[24] Coyne A. The relationship between cognitive impairment and elder abuse. In: Tatara T, editor. Findings of five elder abuse studies. Washington, DC: National Agency Resource Center on Elder Abuse; 1991. p. 23–50.

[25] Coyne AC, Reichman WE, Berbig LJ. The relationship between dementia and elder abuse. Am J Psychiatry 1993;150(4):643–6.

[26] Dyer CB, Pavlick VN, Pace-Murphy K, et al. The high prevalence of depression and dementia in elder abuse and neglect. J Am Geriatr Soc 2000;48(2):205–8.

[27] Haley W, Coleton J. Alzheimer's disease: special issues in elder abuse and neglect. J Elder Abuse Negl 1992;4(4):71–85.

[28] Hamel M, Gold D, Andres D, et al. Predictors and consequences of aggressive behavior by community based dementia patients. Gerontologist 1990;30:206–11.

[29] Moon A, Williams O. Perceptions of elder abuse and help seeking pattern among African American, Caucasian American and Korean-American women. Gerontologist 1993;33: 376–85.

[30] Paveza GJ, Cohen D, Eisdorfer C, et al. Severe family violence and Alzheimer's disease: prevalence and risk factors. Gerontologist 1992;32(4):493–7.

[31] Pepper C, Oakar MR. Elder abuse: an estimation of a hidden problem. In: H. S. C. o. A. US House of Representatives, editor. Washington, D.C.: US Government Printing Office; 1981.

[32] Ryden MB. Aggressive behavior in persons with dementia who live in the community. Alzheimer Dis Assoc Disord 1988;2:342–55.

[33] Steinmetz SK. Duty bound: elder abuse and family care. Volume 166. Newbury Park (CA): Sage Publications; 1988.

[34] VandeWeerd C, Paveza G. Identification of risk factors associated with negative conflict resolution style in Alzheimer's family caregivers. Paper presented at the 55th Annual Scientific Meeting of the Gerontological Society of America. Boston, November 25, 2002.

[35] VandeWeerd C, Paveza G. Verbal mistreatment and Alzheimer's disease. Paper presented at the 57th Annual Scientific Meeting of the Gerontological Society of America. Washington, DC, November 20, 2004.

[36] Wolf R, Pillemer K. Helping elderly victims. The reality of elder abuse. New York: Columbia University Press; 1989.

[37] Fulmer T. Elder mistreatment. Annual Review of Nursing Research 1994;12:51–64.

[38] Pillemer K, Suitor JJ. Violence and violent feelings: what causes them among family caregivers? Journal of Gerontology: Social Sciences 1992;47(4):S165–72.

[39] Reis M, Nahmiash D. Abuse of seniors: personality, stress and other indicators. J Ment Health Aging 1997;3(3):337–56.

[40] Anetzberger G, Korbin J, Austin C. Alcoholism and elder abuse. J Interpers Violence 1994;9(2):184–93.

[41] Bristowe E, Collins J. Family mediated abuse of non-institutionalized frail elderly men and women living in British Colombia. J Elder Abuse Negl 1989;1(1):45–64.

[42] Gioglio G, Blakemore P. Elder abuse in New Jersey: the knowledge and experience of abuse among older New Jerseyans. Trenton (NJ): Division on Aging; 1982.

[43] Kosberg J, Garcia J. Common and unique themes on elder abuse from a world wide perspective. Journal of Elder Abuse and Neglect 1995;6(3/4):183–97.

[44] The National Committee on Elder Abuse. The National Elder Abuse Incidence Study (Final Report). Washington, D.C.: The Administration on Aging (DHHS); 1998.

[45] Pillemer K, Finklenhorn D. The prevalence of elder abuse: a random sample survey. The Gerontologist 1988;28:51–7.

[46] Vinton L. An exploratory study of self-neglectful elderly. J Gerontol Soc Work 1992;18 (1/2):55–67.

[47] Wolf RS, Godkin MA, Pillemer K. Maltreatment of the elderly: a comparative analysis. Pride Institute of Long Term Health Care 1986;5(4):10–7.

[48] Cohen D, Luchins D, Eisdorfer C, et al. Caring for relatives with Alzheimer's disease: the mental health risks to spouses, adult children and other family caregivers. Behavior, Health and Aging 1990;1(3):171–82.

[49] Cohen D, Paveza G, Eisdorfer C. Predicting caregiver burden and depression. Gerontologist 1997;37(Special Issue 1):33–9.

[50] Ruskin PE, Talbott JA, editors. Aging and posttraumatic stress disorder. Washington, D.C: American Psychiatric Press, Inc.; 1996.

[51] Wolf RS, Pillemer KA. The older battered woman: wives and mothers compared. J Ment Health Aging 1997;3(3):325–36.

[52] Flaherty A, Raia P. Beyond risk protection and Alzheimer's disease. J Elder Abuse Negl 1994;6(2):75–93.

[53] Gallagher D, Wrabetz A, Lovett S, et al. Depression and other negative affects in family caregivers. In: Light E, Lebowitz B, editors. Alzheimer's disease treatment and family stress: directions for research. New York: Hemisphere; 1990. p. 218–24.

[54] Haley W, Levin E, Brown S, et al. Psychological, social, and health consequences of caring for a relative with senile dementia. J Am Geriatr Soc 1987;35:405–11.

[55] Kiecolt-Glaser J, Glaser R. Caregiving, mental health, and immune function in Alzheimer's disease treatment and family stress: directions for Research. DHHS Publication (ADM) 89–1569. Washington, DC: US government printing office; 1989.

[56] Podnieks E, Pillemer K, Nicholson J. National Survey of Abuse of Elderly in Canada. Ryerson Polytechnical Institute. Toronto; 1990.

[57] Bendik M. Reaching the breaking point: dangers of the mistreatment in elder caregiving situations. J Elder Abuse Negl 1992;4(3):39–59.

[58] Livtin S. Status transitions and future outlook as determinants of conflict: the caregiver's and care-receiver's perspective. Gerontologist 1992;32:68–76.

[59] Barer BM. The Relationship between homebound older people and their home care worker. J Gerontol Soc Work 1992;19:129–47.

[60] Fulmer TT, O'Malley TA. Inadequate care of the elderly: a health care perspective on abuse and neglect. New York: Springer Publishing Company; 1987.

[61] Rosenblatt DE. Reporting the mistreatment of older adults: the role of physicians. J Am Geriatr Soc 1996;44:65–70.

[62] Pillemer KA, Wolf RS, editors. Elder abuse: conflict in the family. Dover (MA): Auburn House; 1986.

[63] Easterly R, Macpherson R, Richards H, et al. Assaults on professional careers of elderly people. BMJ 1993;307:845–52.

[64] American Medical Association. Diagnostic and Treatment Guidelines on Elder Abuse and Neglect. AA25: 96–7:4M:12/96.

[65] Ahmad M, Lachs M. Elder abuse and neglect: what physicians can and should do. Cleve Clin J Med 2002;69(10):801–8.

[66] Reis M, Nahmiash D. Validation of the indicators of abuse (IOA) screen. Gerontologist 1998;38(4):471–80.

[67] Hwalek MA, Sengstock MC. Hwalek-Sengstock Elder Abuse Screening Test Revised. J Appl Gerontol 1986;5(2):153–73.

[68] Lachs MS, Williams C, O'Brien S, et al. Risk factors for reported elder abuse and neglect: a nine -year observational cohort study. Gerontologist 1997;37(4):469–74.

[69] Fulmer T, Street S, Carr K. Abuse of the elderly: screening and detection. J Emerg Nurs 1984;10(3):131–40.

[70] Brown M, Dehne D. Preventing elder abuse by enhancing caregiver interventions for people with dementia. 2002. Available at: http://www.onpea.org?Strategy/Communication/conferrence02/browndehne.pdf. Accessed July 14, 2005.

[71] Toesland RW, Labvecque MS, Gobel ST. Therapeutic processes in professional and peer counseling of family caregivers to frail elderly. Social Work 1992;37(92):345–51.

[72] Cummings J, Frank J, Cherry D, et al. Guidelines for managing Alzheimer's disease: part II. Treatment. Am Fam Physician 2002;65(12):2263–72.

[73] Craig R, Chow H, Greenbaum M, et al. How well are clinicians following dementia practice guidelines? Alzheimers Disease and Associated Disorder 2002;16(1):15–23.

[74] Gruman, Stern & Caro, 1997.

[75] Pittaway E, Westhues A. The prevalence of elder abuse and neglect of older adults who access health and social services in London, Ontario, Canada. J Elder Abuse Negl 1993;5(4):77–93.

[76] McGhee J. The vulnerability of elderly consumers. Int J Aging Hum Dev 1983;17(3): 223–46.
[77] Pillemer KA, Moore DW. Abuse of patients in nursing homes: findings from a survey of staff. Gerontologist 1989;29(3):314–20.
[78] Board of Children, Youth and Families (US), Committee on the Training Needs of Health Professionals to Respond to Family Violence. In: Cohen F, Salmon ME, Stobo JD, editors. Confronting chronic neglect: the education and training of health professionals on family violence. Washington, DC: National Academies Press; 2002.

Nurs Clin N Am 41 (2006) 57–81

NURSING CLINICS
OF NORTH AMERICA

ELSEVIER
SAUNDERS

Application of the Progressively Lowered Stress Threshold Model Across the Continuum of Care

Marianne Smith, PhD(c), ARNP, CS[a],*,
Geri Richards Hall, PhD, ARNP, CNS, FAAN[b],
Linda Gerdner, PhD, RN[c], Kathleen C. Buckwalter, PhD, RN[d]

[a]University of Iowa College of Nursing, 400 NB, 50 Newton Road, Iowa City, IA 52242, USA
[b]University of Iowa College of Nursing and Medicine, 446 NB, 50 Newton Road, Iowa City, IA 52242, USA
[c]University of Minnesota School of Nursing, 5-160 Weaver-Densford Hall, 308 Harvard Street Southeast East, Minneapolis, MN 55455, USA
[d]University of Iowa College of Nursing 482 NB, 50 Newton Road, Iowa City, IA 52242-1121, USA

OVERVIEW OF THE PROGRESSIVELY LOWERED STRESS THRESHOLD MODEL

Over the last two decades, increasing attention has been paid to the nature of behavioral symptoms in dementia. Early notions that all behaviors were an inevitable component of cognitive impairment have all but disappeared in the face of evidence that diverse personal, social, and environmental factors regularly act as antecedents to behavioral and psychologic symptoms of dementia (BPSD) [1]. The quality of care provided to persons with dementia has been advanced through nursing care conceptual models that explain antecedents to BPSD and, in turn, offer specific interventions to promote comfort and optimal function.

One such model, the Progressively Lowered Stress Threshold (PLST) model of care, was first described in the literature in 1987 [2]. In the years since, the PLST model has provided an important framework for the education of formal and family caregivers and the development of individualized plans of care for individuals with dementia [3,4]. This combination of aims, education of caregivers and personalized care, focuses on supporting the person with dementia in a "prosthetic manner"—that is, helping them to use remaining skills and abilities while minimizing the risk of unnecessarily triggering negative reactions and responses by adapting the environment and care routines. The model is appealing to caregivers (who often are stressed themselves and understand the concepts well) and is grounded in theories about confusion, aging,

*Corresponding author. E-mail address: Marianne-smith@uiowa.edu (M. Smith).

0029-6465/06/$ – see front matter
doi:10.1016/j.cnur.2005.09.006
nursing.theclinics.com

ARCHBISHOP ALEMANY LIBRARY
DOMINICAN UNIVERSITY
SAN RAFAEL, CALIFORNIA 94901

SMITH, HALL, GERDNER, ET AL

dementia, stress and coping, and client-centered care [5–9]. This article provides a brief overview of the PLST model and describes how the theoretic model may be applied across the continuum of care by using a case vignette to illustrate common problems and care solutions that are guided by the principles of care.

Progressively Lowered Stress Threshold

In brief, the PLST model suggests that four clusters of BPSD are observed in dementia. Three clusters of behavior are related to losses that occur as dementia progresses, including impairments in cognitive, affective, and planning abilities. The fourth cluster, called PLST, includes an array of behaviors that emerge when environmental demands, external or internal, exceed the person's ability to cope and adapt. Symptoms in the PLST cluster, such as agitation, night wakening, late-day confusion, and combative behaviors are hypothesized to be stress related.

According to the model, persons with dementia increasingly are less able to manage stress as the disease progresses. Their stress threshold or capacity to tolerate stress is reduced, resulting first in anxious behaviors and attempts to reduce stress, such as demanding to leave an area. If the stress is unrelieved, behaviors which are characterized by cognitive and social inaccessibility [5] and reduced ability to function (eg, agitation) are likely to emerge (Fig. 1). Of equal importance, triggers for stress take many forms for persons with dementia, including: fatigue; changes in routine, caregiver, or environment; internal or external demands that exceed the person's ability to function; multiple and competing stimuli; affective responses by the person with dementia to his/her perception of lost abilities; and physical stress, such as illness, discomfort (eg, hunger, full bladder), adverse reactions to medications, and pain [10]. As shown in Fig. 2, caregivers can facilitate more adaptive behavior by regulating stress for the person with dementia and by intervening when anxiety-related symptoms appear.

The PLST model proposes six essential principles of care. Each principle offers direction for an array of general interventions that are then further

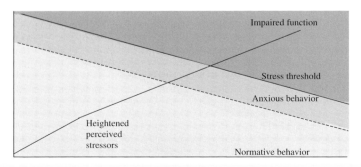

Fig. 1. Stress threshold in a patient with Alzheimer's disease and related dementia.

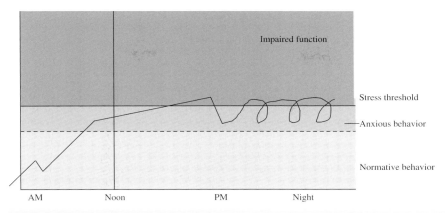

Fig. 2. Effects of stress during a 24-hour day.

individualized to assure that the unique needs of each person are addressed. Many illustrations of general interventions are available in professional and training literature today [4,10–12], including but not limited to the examples described below.

Maximize safe function by supporting all losses in a "prosthetic" manner
Caregivers can help the person with dementia be successful by changing routines and approaches and by keeping stress at a manageable level. Seemingly "simple" adjustments help persons with dementia use their remaining abilities, thus promoting self worth and dignity. General interventions include things like using a calm, consistent routine, and avoiding attempts to "reason" with the person, asking them to "try harder," or trying to teach them new skills. Supporting lost abilities also involves use of familiar routines and an unhurried pace, alternating high and low stimulus activities, limiting choices to ones the person can make, and planned rest periods to reduce stress levels. Reducing stimuli when stress reactions occur (eg, reducing noise, moving to a quiet space, and checking for physical stressors, such as hunger, pain, or wetness) allows the person to regain "control" and return to baseline.

Provide unconditional positive regard
Showing respect for the person and the long life he/she has lived is exemplified in communication strategies and allowing the person to use intact skills and abilities. One-to-one communication methods include use of simple and understandable language, appropriate nonverbal gestures for emphasis, gentle touch to reassure, elimination of "you are wrong" messages (eg, "No, you live here now" in response to wanting to go home), and use of distraction or acceptance rather than confrontation. Likewise, helping persons with dementia perform daily activities on their own by giving simple instructions and cueing, instead of taking over and "doing things to" the person, promotes self worth.

Use behaviors to gauge activity and stimulation levels

Expressions of rising anxiety, such as demanding to leave, walking away, or withdrawing from activity, should be respected (eg, do not try to stop the person). Monitoring the situation to identify possible cues to stress reactions and "early" anxious behaviors, such as toe tapping, worried facial expressions, or increased pacing, allows caregivers to intervene before the person escalates into more distressed and uncomfortable behaviors. Teaching caregivers to recognize that abrupt changes in behavior may signal distress and the need for intervention, and to keep careful records of activities and times of day that correlate with increased anxiety or other behavioral symptoms, is often essential to maintaining comfort and function for the person with dementia.

Teach caregivers to "listen" to behaviors

As dementia progresses, the person is less able to use language to express needs and feelings. Teaching caregivers to listen carefully to the spoken words (eg, jargon, repetitive questions) and behavioral expressions (eg, rummaging or pacing that may be seeking something) may reduce stress reactions when needs are not met. Family caregivers, in particular, are often able to "decipher" seemingly bizarre words or behaviors that are grounded in the person's past experiences or routines.

Modify the environment to support losses

In conjunction with changing routines, the goals of maintaining safety and keeping stress at a manageable level regularly involves adapting the physical and social environments. Assessing the physical environment for possible barriers or hazards (eg, steps, scatter rugs, inadequate lighting) and objects that may be misused as a result of impairments (eg, household cleansers, guns, power tools, stove, automobile) is essential to making needed adaptations. Taking down pictures, drawing drapes to reduce reflections, reducing clutter, and turning off television may reduce misinterpretations that lead to delusions. Function may be promoted by adding signage to promote way-finding, cues to promote orientation, and color contrast to enhance visualization of needed objects (eg, toilet, steps). Intermittent evaluation of visual-spatial deficits (eg, clock drawing test) and driving safety, and use of identification bracelets, are additional safety considerations.

Provide on-going assistance to formal and informal caregivers

In light of the considerable responsibility often assumed by family members and other day-to-day caregivers, ongoing assessment of their needs and responses is essential. Assessment parameters often include their understanding of dementia, physical and mental health (particularly depression), objective and subjective levels of burden, conflict between family members, and sources of support and assistance. Referrals for concrete assistance in providing care, support groups, educational programs, and other community resources help provide needed support. Teaching caregivers to recognize their own limits, seek help for negative feelings like anger, and engage in stress-reducing activities themselves, helps sustain their ongoing therapeutic approaches.

The PLST model is recommended as a framework for devising nonpharmacologic interventions for persons with dementia across living environments [13] and has been applied and evaluated in various settings, including home care [13,14], nursing homes [11], special care units [15,16], hospitals [17], and adult day health centers (ADHC). The usefulness of the PLST model, however, is perhaps best understood through the use of clinical care vignettes that illustrate key care principles in these diverse care settings. Thus, this article applies the PLST principles to the care of "Vera Detweiler" as she moves from one care setting to another in response to her changing levels of health, social support, and care needs. Although Vera is an amalgamation of persons with dementia, the services described and processes involved in her care depict real programs of care that are increasingly available to persons with dementia. Brief descriptions of novel projects and services on which this vignette is based are provided in endnotes.

Vera Lives at Home

Vera Detweiler is an 83-year-old widow who lives alone in the farm home in which she has resided for over 60 years. After her husband Hans died 10 years ago, Vera's ability to live at home increasingly relied on the support and assistance of her daughter Margaret and son-in-law Dieter, who live on the adjoining farm. Her son Peter, who lived on the coast, handled legal and financial matters, including management of Vera's farm, income, and investments. Margaret and Peter shared power of attorney, which included health care decision-making. Two years ago, Vera was diagnosed with Alzheimer's type dementia after a long and troubling course of changes in her memory, mood, personality, and behavior.

An outgoing and social woman throughout her life, Vera concealed her memory impairment for an extended period but experienced one "mishap" after another—in her kitchen, home, yard; while walking to visit a nearby neighbor; and driving. Strange ideas, including the beliefs that "little people" were in her house at night, that an "old woman" was spying on her, and that her food was being poisoned, became more frequent and troubling. Self and home-care deficits, including failure to bathe, groom, and change clothes regularly, or to wash dishes and clean the house, were completely out of character, as Vera had always been meticulous in her appearance and home maintenance. The family suspected Vera was not eating as her clothing hung loosely. Even more disturbing were bouts of irritable and angry behavior, usually in response to Margaret pushing her mother to "keep things up" or explain unfamiliar word or phrases, which were contrary to Vera's usual even-tempered nature.

In response, Margaret became overly protective of her mother, whereas Peter dismissed his sister's observations and actions as exaggerated, "controlling," and unnecessary. After considerable family turmoil and disagreement about the nature of Vera's problems, her long-time family physician referred her to a comprehensive health center where an interdisciplinary assessment was conducted, the diagnosis of probable Alzheimer's disease was derived, and numerous community care referrals were made. As part of the assessment, a nurse went to Vera's home to perform the Assessment for Risk of Living Alone (ARLA).[1] Based on the PLST model, the ARLA identifies those observations that are emergent, semi-emergent, and nonemergent. The ARLA assists professionals to determine goals for care and to predict how quickly additional interventions are needed based on the degree of urgency identified [18].

Substantial educational, supportive, and health-related services provided under the supervision of a dementia care nurse manager (DCNM)[2] were needed to sustain Vera at home. Using PLST principles, the DCNM helped the family adapt Vera's home to promote function and safety, modify routines to promote autonomy and comfort, and arrange for additional services to relieve Margaret and Dieter's burden and stress. Because Peter had long resisted the idea that his mother was seriously impaired, and thus opposed paying for formal services, the nurse manager encouraged an extended visit. Staying with his mother for two weeks while Margaret and Dieter were on vacation increased Peter's awareness of Vera's declining abilities and helped him see the value of alternative and supportive care services.

Because Vera lived outside a wealthy metropolitan community that was committed to providing home-based services for older adults,[3] the DCNM was able to assemble needed services quickly. Arrangements were made for Vera to attend the ADHC four days per week. The ADHC provided on-site personal cares, including bathing and grooming, and two meals daily (breakfast and lunch), medication administration, and an array of medical, social, and leisure activities. Of importance, the day center employed gardening and cooking as therapeutic interventions, making the transition to the center an easy one for Vera. Center staff were all trained in the PLST model and the facility offered a lower stimulus dementia-specific unit, thus assuring the care plan developed by the DCNM and family was followed.[4] On the other three days, a home health aid was hired to spend four hours a day with Vera to assist with personal cares and grocery shopping, administer medications, prepare lunch and a light supper to be eaten later, and initiate activities, such as gardening, walking together, and having Vera rest after lunch. After Margaret and Peter cleaned

---

[1]The assessment process described here was developed as a component of "Building a Seamless Dementia-Specific Service Delivery System for Rural Iowa," Grant 90AZ2366, an Administration on Aging Alzheimer's disease demonstration project awarded to the Iowa Department of Elder Affairs, directed by co-investigators Drs. Janet K. Specht and Geri R. Hall, University of Iowa College of Nursing. Contact Project Director Ann Bossen at ann.bossen@uiowa.edu for more information about the project.

[2]The roles and responsibilities of the dementia care nurse manager (DCNM) described here are consistent with roles of Memory Loss Nurse Specialists in the project "Building a Seamless Dementia-Specific Service Delivery System for Iowa" described previously.

[3]The services described here represent the array that is available to older adults living in rural communities outside the Iowa City and Cedar Rapids Communities in Iowa.

[4]Services described here are available at Milestones Adult Day Health Center, a program located in Cedar Rapids, Iowa. Milestones serves an average of 65 older and disabled adults daily, and employs the HEAL (Health, Environment, Arts and Humanities, Lifelong Learning) Model of care. The program has been replicated at Pathways, in Iowa City, Iowa, and Milestones II in Hiawatha, Iowa. Contact jbenson-vorwald@abbe.org for information about the program.

the house, a homemaker was hired to clean and do laundry. Scheduled telephone and in-person visits by a cadre of trusted friends and neighbors provided supplemental assistance to help Vera continue living at home, thus giving Margaret and Dieter additional relief from caregiving. Key elements of the care plan developed to sustain Vera in her farm home are outlined in Table 1.

Although Vera continued to decline, the DCNM assured that services were adapted to meet her changing needs and that her safety was maintained. Knowing how Vera loved her flower and vegetable gardens (now maintained with help from church volunteers), her many cats, bird watching, and just rocking on the front porch, Margaret and Peter supported all changes to help sustain their mother at home. At the same time, Vera's adult children were aging themselves. Dieter's health was failing, and Margaret worried that their time together might be limited. After considerable discussion, the couple decided to take an extended vacation in their motor home, a lifetime retirement dream that was deterred after Hans died and Vera became increasingly dependent.

Without Margaret and Dieter's daily visits and monitoring, everyone agreed that Vera would be safer in the town's newly constructed assisted living facility (ALF). Because Margaret and Dieter planned to travel throughout the fall but return home before the holidays, arrangements were made for Vera to be placed in the ALF as a "respite" client.

Vera Moves to Assisted Living

As identified in the PLST model, changes in the environment, caregivers, and daily routines often trigger behaviors that impair function and comfort. The DCMN recognized that all three would come into play with the move to institutional care. Thus, substantial preparations were made to reduce relocation stress and assure a smooth transition from Vera's home to the assisted living apartment where she would live during the fall months. Important pieces of furniture, personal and household possessions, and hobby-related activities were assembled to assure her new location was as homelike as possible. The DCNM collaborated with family and staff of the ALF to develop a care plan that mimicked routines that had been successful at home. Arrangements were made for the homemaker and home health aide, who now knew Vera quite well, to continue their services on a reduced basis in the apartment. Likewise, Vera's participation in the adult day health program was continued. The DCNM provided the ALF staff with in-service education on the PLST model, including a discussion session in which the care principles were applied to common problems related to relocation from home, such as elopement related to "wanting to go home." To the extent possible, Vera was included in all discussions and decision-making, and a summary of the process was recorded in a visual "reminder" book that contained pictures of Vera's home, family members, the new ALF, and ended with pictures reinforcing that Vera would be returning to her home and family. Videotapes and audiotapes of Margaret and Dieter were made before their departure in anticipation that Vera would miss their daily visits and would worry about their absence. Favorite fall activities

Table 1
Progressively lowered stress threshold care plan for Vera's home care

PLST principle	Identified problems/needs	Interventions

Maintain safe function by supporting losses in a prosthetic manner.	Self-care deficits: bathing, grooming, changing clothes; weight loss evidenced by loose clothing
	
	Home-care deficits: home maintenance and safety issues
		• Develop and maintain a routine to assure appropriate supervision and supportive services;
		  ✔ ADHC 4 day/week
		  ✔ HHA 3 days a week
		  ✔ Homemaker services weekly
		  ✔ Daily phone calls (rotation of family, formal and informal caregivers)
		  ✔ Daily visits (rotation of family, formal and informal caregivers)
		• Monitor grooming and hygiene; encourage/cue use of daily routines at home and ADHC.
		• Maintain a supply of nutritious, fresh finger foods, salads, sandwiches, snacks, and cold drinks are available in home refrigerator to supplement scheduled meals at ADHC and home.
		• Provide a large-print month-long calendar that outlines daily routines as a visual reminder.
		• Administer medications: 4 days at ADHC; 3 days by HHA
		• Secure an OT assessment of possible home adaptations to promote functional capacity; implement suggestions and re-evaluate in 3 months.

Provide unconditional positive regard.	Family knowledge deficits: dementia processes, communication methods, behavioral symptoms, and PLST principles
	
	Community caregiver knowledge deficits: communication methods, behavioral symptoms, and PLST principles
		• Teach family and other caregivers about loss of abilities in dementia, PLST principles, and communication methods
		• Specific strategies include:
		  ✔ Avoid "you are wrong" messages. Do not "correct" false beliefs such as seeing "little people", food being poisoned, or someone spying on her.
		  ✔ Offer concern for her distress, then attempt to distract to more positive thoughts or activities: review of pictures/discussion of flowers, cats, birds, weather, crops, and recent events.
		  ✔ If she becomes upset or angry, either agree, apologize, play "dumb," or suggest you discuss it tomorrow.

Use anxiety and avoidance to gauge activity and stimulation levels.	Potential stress reactions: irritability and anger in response to being "pushed" to use lost abilities	• Monitor Vera's behavior to identify cues to possible stress reactions:
		  ✓ Note associations between reactions and events in the behavior log.
		  ✓ List possible triggers (physical, social, personal environment).
		  ✓ Note responses to interventions used to reduce anger or irritability.
		• Do not "push" if Vera becomes more irritable, anxious, or unhappy with the topic or issue at hand.
		• Invite/coax/encourage a "time out" if a reaction occurs; useful distractions include having a sweet snack, finding the cat, walking out to check on the garden, and listening to her music tapes.

Teach caregivers to "listen" to the person with dementia.	Language impairment: use of unfamiliar words and jargon that family do not understand	• Record "jargon" or other unusual words and phrases that Vera commonly uses.
		• Note interventions used to "solve problems" related to unknown word/jargon and success of same in behavioral log.
		• Ask "why do you ask?" if Vera repeatedly asks the same question.
		• Evaluate possible unmet needs based on her usual routine and the time of day; offer supportive interventions as appropriate:
		  ✓ Food, fluids for hunger/thirst
		  ✓ Activity/distraction (eg, walking, garden, cats/birds)

Modify the environment to support losses.	Safety issues: mishaps in the kitchen, home and yard, walking to the neighbors, and driving Paranoia: television stimulated delusion of "little people" in the house; reflection of self-perceived as "old woman" spying on her; spoiled, malodorous food perceived as "poison"	• Safety-proof the house and yard (eg, remove throw rugs, disable the oven, use color contrast to promote accurate visual input on steps and in bathroom; lock up insecticides, herbicides, and cleaning products; place a fence as a barrier between the yard and woods; mow a walking path to neighbor's house; disable the car). • Monitor use of identification bracelet (eg, Vera does not remove); keep Safe Return information up-to-date. • Monitor and record reactions to safety interventions applied (eg, climbing the fence); identify new misinterpretations/potential hazards. • Assure all food is fresh and edible to reduce risk that spoiled food triggers thoughts of being poisoned. • Cover/remove mirrors, close drapes at night to reduce risk that she misinterprets her own image as an intruder.

(continued on next page)

Table 1
(continued)

PLST principle	Identified problems/needs	Interventions
Provide on-going education, support, care and assistance with problem-solving to caregivers.	Family knowledge deficits: daughter is "over protective"; son is "denying" problems Family respite: Margaret and Dieter are providing all care needs	• Encourage family to participate in live and on-line support groups. • Reassure family that conflict is normal; encourage information gathering and discussion of perceptions. • Reinforce teaching on disease progression and PLST model. • Reinforce need for supportive services, respite, and family's need to care for themselves. • Encourage family to seek and use health services on a regular basis. • Monitor and reinforce support and assistance provided by neighbors and close friends

Abbreviations: ADHC, adult day health center; HHA, home health aide; OT, occupational therapy.

were reviewed with staff and incorporated into the care plan as a means to entertain, support, and distract Vera as the need arose. Likewise, care plans at the adult day health program were adapted to help assure continued involvement in meaningful activities in the center's gardens, including plans to engage Vera in freezing produce, as she would have done with Margaret at home.

All parties recognized that unexpected social or health-related problems might emerge during Vera's 12-week stay. Thus, key information about Vera, including her health history, mental status, and legal decision-makers, were put in an envelope and placed in her chart to assure all relevant records were immediately available if needed. Because Margaret and Dieter anticipated that they would not be available by telephone during part of their trip, the DCNM was designated as the "first contact," with back-up from Peter, who shared power of attorney for health care decisions. Although the ALF had a small outdoor area, arrangements were made for a volunteer to take Vera walking outdoors as she often did at home. Finally, adjustments were made in the information provided to the Safe Return[5] program to assure that records were up-to-date about Vera's current appearance, living arrangements, and contact persons.

Despite efforts to promote Vera's adaptation to her new surroundings, once at the ALF she required constant reassurance that this "new home" was a temporary one. She repeatedly asked to "go home," and often was found checking doors in the evening. Her appetite, which was usually robust, diminished and she began to refuse foods that she regularly enjoyed. Changes in her care plan were undertaken to offer structured activities at times she typically became restless (eg, in the evening) and to assure that small meals and fluids, including familiar German snacks such as eier-apel-toast, were provided more often throughout the day. Refer to Table 2 [19] to review key components of Vera's care plan at the ALF.

After a week, Vera began to settle into her new routine; however, in early October when decorations and activities related to Halloween increasingly became the focus throughout the ALF, staff observed that Vera began spending more time alone in her apartment. In turn, opportunities for nutrition and hydration were reduced, "odd" thoughts returned, and attempts to leave the facility increased. Although most staff were aware of Vera's exit-seeking behaviors, a visiting nursery school teacher left an exterior door in the kitchen ajar "for a few minutes" while she brought in party food and Vera left the facility. Wearing no outerwear, the fall wind soon became overwhelming. She was later found by the rescue crew in a ditch only a few blocks from the facility, but obscured from view by the tall grass where she fell. Vera was transported

---

[5]Safe Return, a nationwide program of the Alzheimer's Association, provides assistance 24 hours a day, seven days a week, when a person with dementia wanders and becomes lost locally or far from home. The program requires a one-time enrollment fee and provides identification products to promote identification and return of the person with dementia (eg, identification bracelet, necklace, and iron-on clothing labels). See http://www.alz.org/safereturn/ for additional information about the program.

Table 2
Progressively lowered stress threshold care plan for assisted living care

PLST principle	Identified problems/needs	Interventions

Maintain safe function by supporting losses in a prosthetic manner.	Relocation stress: unfamiliar staff/residents
	Relocation stress: unfamiliar routines
	Continuing self-care deficits
	Continuing activity needs
	Appetite/sleep disturbance
		• Staff training on PLST model; questions re: care should be directed to the shift supervisor; contact the DCNM for clarification and assistance as needed
		• Promote orientation to the facility, staff, and routines by using gentle orientation and information-sharing:
		  ✓ All caregivers introduce themselves each time they interact with Vera.
		  ✓ Introduce her to other residents, then continue to cue her about their names and possible relationship to her (eg, used to farm near her; was in the same church).
		  ✓ Volunteer information about the facility and routines to reassure her.
		  ✓ Always knock and wait for a reply before entering her apartment; gently cue about van arrival and other events activities.
		  ✓ Maintain and refer to the large print calendar that outlines her routines.
		• Continue personal care by known care providers to minimize disruption to routines and promote continuity:
		  ✓ ADHC 4 days/week
		  ✓ HHA 3 days/week, 2 hours per day: bathing, grooming, cue to eat lunch at facility, outings as desired
		  ✓ Homemaker 1 day/week, 2 hours: apartment cleaning and shopping
		• Encourage nutrition and hydration:
		  ✓ Gently remind and cue her about meal times; limit food selection to foods she likes and eats (see list in kitchen).
		  ✓ Offer/cue to eat snacks throughout the day; offer juice at least 3 times/day (favorites: apple, cranberry).
		• Promote usual sleep/wake routines: routinely close her drapes at night, and open in the morning to cue rising and sleeping patterns (and avoid misinterpretations).

Provide unconditional positive regard.	Facility staff knowledge deficits: PLST principles	• Apply PLST home-care plan principles; additional interventions include:
		  ✔ Do not argue if Vera wants to "go home"; gently remind her that she is "visiting"; attempt to distract with tapes, videos, or memory book.
		  ✔ Invite to kitchen or garden area, asking for her "help" to redirect.
		• Apply all strategies used in Home Health Care Plan

Use anxiety and avoidance to gauge activity and stimulation levels.	Ongoing risk of stress reactions	
Teach caregivers to "listen" to the person with dementia.	Ongoing language impairment	• Apply all strategies used in Home Health Care Plan

Modify the environment to support losses.	Loneliness: social and safety needs related to the absence of daily family contacts
	
	Elopement risk
		• Promote continuity and familiarity by using and discussing personal possessions during care (eg, pictures, bedding, recliner, plants, and other items from home).
		• Encourage usual activities: gardening, walking, food preparation (ADHC, HHA, facility staff).
		• Safeguard against elopement risk: maintain use of identification bracelet; update Safe Return records; monitor doors when visitors arrive/exit.
		• Engage in activities after evening meal or when pacing or exit-seeking behaviors are observed; rotation of therapeutic intervention includes:
		  ✔ Individualized music interventions [19]: audio tapes of Vera's favorite records played in her room
		  ✔ Pet therapy: facility cat preferred; dog is acceptable alternative
		  ✔ Food preparation: favorite is preparing/baking cookies
		  ✔ Telephone support: list of trusted friends, neighbors who provide reassurance and support is located in bedside stand drawer
		  ✔ Avoid walking outdoors after evening meal; reserve for mid-day activity in full daylight; gardens preferred area

(continued on next page)

Table 2
(continued)

PLST principle	Identified problems/needs	Interventions
Provide on-going education, support, care and assistance with problem-solving to caregivers.	Facility staff knowledge deficits: Vera's longstanding patterns and habits Availability of a legal decision-maker	• Refer to comprehensive social history in chart if questions arise about habits, preferences, and behaviors. • Contact DCNM if questions about care plan arise; see numbers on face page of chart. • If change of status or untoward incident, notify DCNM, son Peter, and primary care physician simultaneously; see numbers on face page of chart. • Note: voice messages left on daughter Margaret's cell phone may not be retrieved due to travel conflicts

Abbreviation: HHA, home health aide.

to the local hospital, evaluated in the emergency department, and admitted to the medical unit for treatment of hypothermia, dehydration, and delirium.

Challenges During Vera's Brief Hospitalization

Existing physical frailty related to recent nutrition and hydration changes were further aggravated by nearly two hours of exposure in the chilly fall weather. Acute confusion caused by delirium overlapped onto Vera's existing dementia, causing substantial impairment in all aspects of cognitive and physical function. Disorientation, psychomotor agitation, and sleep disturbance were all pronounced, making administration of needed intravenous fluids difficult, and resulting in use of wrist restraints. Soon after, paranoid delusions that medical personnel were trying to kill her, emerged and were treated with antipsychotic medication. Because of Vera's existing diagnosis of dementia, medical staff erroneously presumed Vera was incapable of becoming reoriented, failed to provide her with needed information about her health and circumstances, and instead relied heavily on "as needed" medications and restraints to sedate and "control" her. To monitor her "aberrant" behaviors, she was placed in a room near the busy (and noisy) nurses' station where a ward clerk could visualize her continuously. From the moment of admission, the plan was to "discharge to a secure nursing facility" to assure her safety needs.

The DCNM, now acting as the proxy decision-maker in the family's absence, demanded a care conference to review Vera's current needs and treatments. She skillfully argued on behalf of making changes to reduce the need for physical and chemical restraints and for moving Vera to a room where the level of stimulation could be regulated more easily. After providing a condensed inservice on the PLST model to staff at change of shift, she engaged the help of Vera's newly assigned "primary nurse" in communication principle for her care throughout the team. Relevant components of earlier care plans, from home and ALF care, were placed in the chart for reference and a new care plan was developed in cooperation with the DCNM. To increase appropriate input, items from Vera's home and apartment were immediately brought to the hospital room, audiotapes of family voices were played, picture books were provided to help reorient her, and a rotating schedule of visitors, who knew Vera and the situation well and served as "sitters," was arranged. Refer to Table 3 [20–24] to review the PLST Care Plan for Hospitalization.

Over the brief course of hospitalization, the DCNM worked with the medical team to enhance their skills in dementia management, using the PLST as a framework, and providing considerable supportive literature to validate her requests. With supportive input from Vera's long-time family physician, changes to the treatment plan were made, with the important exception of the discharge plan. Despite arguments that Vera could again be safe in the ALF with additional supportive services, the medical team persuasively argued in favor of a "brief" admission to skilled nursing care to assure that Vera was "medically stable." The benefits of 24-hour nursing supervision and rehabilitation services were considered essential until the delirium subsided and

Table 3
Progressively lowered stress threshold care plan during hospitalization

PLST principle	Identified problems/needs	Interventions

Maintain safe function by supporting losses in a prosthetic manner.	Change in medical status: hypothermia, dehydration, nutritional deficits, bruised ankle secondary to falling
	
	Change in mental status: delirium secondary to medical problems and relocation
	
	Symptom management: disorientation, psychomotor agitation, sleep disturbance, paranoid delusions
	
	Iatrogenic health problems: use of chemical and physical restraints
		• Apply principles used prior to hospitalization to reduce behavioral symptoms observed in patient:
		  ✓ Refer to educational materials provided by patient's DCNM during inservice for additional information about patient's care and rational for interventions.
		  ✓ Contact DCMN if questions or problems related to behavioral symptoms and confusion; numbers are on face sheet in chart and social history.
		  ✓ Refer to prior care plan (in chart) for additional information about history, preferences, and successful approaches used with patient.
		• Conduct physical assessments at least Q shift; vital signs at least Q 2 hours × 2 days.
		• Maintain continuity by assigning consistent staff to patient throughout hospitalization (eg, do not rotate staff assignments if possible).
		• Patient is unlikely to report pain; use behavioral symptoms as barometer for discomfort:
		  ✓ Schedule pain medication administration; use PRN only for breakthrough pain as assessed below.
		  ✓ Monitor pain using PAINAD [20] Q shift and PRN related to movement (eg, daily cares, physical therapy)
		• Assess mental status Q shift and document in flow chart:
		  ✓ Mini Mental State Exam [21]
		  ✓ Confusion Assessment Method [22]
		• Provide gentle, conversational orientation to remind patient of falling, hospitalization, and need for medical care.
		  ✓ Introduce self, offering day, date, time, and place during each interaction.
		  ✓ Provide anticipatory guidance and explanations related to cares and activities.
		• Assess/monitor potential for falling:
		  ✓ Leave bed in lowest position.
		  ✓ Avoid side rails; use half rail only to steady the side patient is using; line other side with pillows.
		  ✓ Use bed alarm at all times.

Provide unconditional positive regard.

Use anxiety and avoidance to gauge activity and stimulation levels.

- ✔ Place walker near bed where patient can see it to cue use.
- Promote oral fluid and food intake:
  - ✔ Serve six small meals per day, following food preference list in chart.
  - ✔ Cue oral intake to exceed 2000 cc days, 1600 cc evenings, 500 cc nights.
  - ✔ Avoid use of foley catheters, IVs, nasogastric tubes.
- Avoid use of physical and chemical restraints:
  - ✔ Use least restrictive restraint method following protocol "Outside the Box: Restraint Alternatives that Work in Acute Care" [23] filed in chart.
  - ✔ Avoid use of antipsychotics and benzodiazepines.
  - ✔ Employ nonpharmacologic interventions used previously to assure, distract, and calm patient; see list of alternatives in Home Health Care Plan filed in chart.
- Continue acetylcholinesterace inhibitor throughout hospitalization and at discharge.
- Apply strategies in Home Health Care Plan and reviewed during inservice.

Staff knowledge deficits: PLST principles

Stress reactions: increased risk cause delirium and relocation

- Monitor type and frequency of behavioral symptoms:
  - ✔ Apply Cohen Mansfield Agitation Inventory [24] as checklist Q shift.
  - ✔ Note associations between care procedures, and other stimuli and behaviors.
  - ✔ Adjust routines and approaches in accordance to patterns observed.
- Apply strategies in Home Health Care Plan and reviewed during inservice.
- Apply strategies in Home Health Care Plan and reviewed during inservice.

Teach caregivers to "listen" to the person with dementia

Ongoing language deficits

Modify the environment to support losses

Over stimulation: room near nurses' station

- Place patient in private room away from busy/noisy areas of unit.
- Encourage use/discussion of familiar personal items provided by home health care team (eg, her pillow, familiar clothing, and family picture).

(continued on next page)

Table 3
(continued)

PLST principle	Identified problems/needs	Interventions
		• Arrange for familiar care providers to visit when increased anxiety is more likely in late afternoon and evening:
		✓Refer to list of nonfamily members who are well-known to patient and willing to assist in chart.
		✓Contact DCMN for additional assistance or information if psychomotor agitation/sleep disturbance persists.
		• Avoid having TV on in room.
		• Use alternative interventions previously employed in Assisted Living Care plan as appropriate: music, review of pictures, ambulation, and telephone support.
		• Request psychiatric consultation and contact DNCM if psychotic symptoms increase or become upsetting to the patient.
Provide on-going education, support, care, and assistance with problem-solving to caregivers.	Staff knowledge deficits	• Apply principles and protocols in Assisted Living Care Plan.
		• Involve DNCM in all discharge planning processes.

Abbreviation: PAINAD, pain assessment in advanced dementia.

laboratory values normalized. Medical staff projected that an additional four weeks of skilled care would assure Vera's return to her prior level of function and, in turn, resolution of residual delirium symptoms that might complicate her care in the ALF or living at home. Although this plan violated earlier family requests to avoid nursing home care "if at all possible," the stance taken by Vera's family physician served as the proverbial "swing vote."

Because a skilled bed was not available in the local community, Vera was discharged to an unfamiliar facility in a larger town nearly 50 miles away. The decision was a difficult one for all involved because supportive services from local community providers were impossible. Vera's care now would rely exclusively on the capabilities of the new, unknown care center and its staff. At the same time, Vera's ongoing physical health needs made it difficult to reject the array of medical services offered. After a brief five days of hospitalization, Vera was transferred again, this time to a skilled nursing facility (SNF) that focused on rehabilitation and return to community living.

Demands of the Skilled Care Facility

Once again the DCNM took a lead role in assuring that appropriate documents were provided to the SNF: from Vera's brief hospitalization, care in the ALF, and plans to return home once Margaret and Dieter returned. She accompanied Vera on the day she was transferred to the facility and requested that a care planning meeting be scheduled as soon as possible to assure that goals, methods, and outcomes for Vera's care were shared and clearly identified. However, the SNF nurse manager was on vacation and no care planning conferences were conducted in her absence. The DCNM was assured that an "interim plan of care" was put in place based on the "information provided" and that a more formal meeting would occur the next week. The interim plan, however, was based on the admission assessment conducted by the newly appointed assistant nurse manager and the faxed discharge plan from the hospital, which included medication orders and goals of care for SNF placement. Written documents mailed to the facility were directed to the nurse manager's office, but were not reviewed in her absence.

Because the primary goal of the hospital's discharge plan was "to return the patient to her prior level of function within four weeks" an aggressive program of reality orientation, nutrition/hydration, and rest alternating with exercise was initiated. The primary focus was on Vera's ability to complete activities of daily living, with little regard to limitations created by her underlying dementia. No attention was paid to her social, recreational, or activity needs which were clearly tied to her functional abilities. Traditional physical therapy (PT) and occupational therapy (OT), along with dietitian services, were enlisted to assure a rehabilitation-oriented care plan was in place when the nurse manager returned the following week.

Challenges created by relocation, unfamiliar staff and physical surroundings, and unrealistic demands for performance soon provoked a series of adverse behavioral reactions. Within a week, Vera began resisting rehabilitation-oriented

Table 4
Progressively lowered stress threshold care plan for the Eden Alternative™ nursing facility

PLST principle	Identified problems/needs	Interventions
Maintain safe function by supporting losses in a prosthetic manner.	Relocation stress: adaptation to new facility and routine; continuing delirium Potential for falls caused by increased autonomy and disease progression. Continuing self-care deficits	• Staff training on PLST model: incorporate principles into care routines: ✓ Refer to home and ALF care plans on file in chart for ideas related to Vera's care. ✓ Refer to training handouts for additional general information about PLST model and care strategies. ✓ Review comprehensive personal and social history (updated on admission) as reference for long-standing habits and patterns of living. • Use nonpharmacologic interventions as an alternative to medication to prevent/reduce behavioral symptoms. ✓ Reinstitute music, pet therapy, simulated presence, horticulture, cooking, and other interventions as distractions. ✓ Escort to outdoor therapeutic gardens, aviary, or facility pet area as needed. ✓ Maintain pain management protocols (eg, PAINAD; scheduled analgesics supplemented with PRN doses prior to potentially uncomfortable daily cares or physical activities). • Promote adaptation and orientation to facility and routines; apply facility protocol: New Resident Orientation: ✓ Provide one-to-one assistance in potentially high-stress situations as needed (eg, finding dining area, meeting other residents, joining activities) until signs of discomfort resolve. ✓ Consistently introduce self; provide anticipatory guidance and explanations for all cares and activities. • Implement fall risk-management program in cooperation with DCMN and family: ✓ Assess Vera monthly or if change in status for fall, risk using standardized tool. ✓ Keep bed in low position without side rails. ✓ Continue PT with goal of maintaining ambulation using her walker; train staff to maintain PT regimen following course of therapy. ✓ If falls occur, substitute a low bed frame. ✓ Make podiatrist appointments monthly for toenail and foot care.

Principle	Need	Intervention

Provide unconditional positive regard.	Unfamiliar staff and routine	✔ Assure that Vera wears shoes with smooth soles, that shoes are in good repair and fit properly.
		• Encourage/cue Vera to participate in personal cares as she is able:
		  ✔ Use method and time Vera prefers (see history for preferences).
		  ✔ Adapt routine if resistance observed and communicate change through shift report.
		  ✔ OT evaluation of functional abilities and needs at admission and monthly for 3 months, as needed.
		• Use standard facility protocol: Promoting Dignity and Respect.

Use anxiety and avoidance to gauge activity and stimulation levels.	Ongoing risk of stress reactions related to unfamiliar facility, staff and routine	• Use facility protocol: New Resident Orientation (see above). • Use facility protocol: Behavior Monitoring.
Teach caregivers to "listen" to the person with dementia.	Unfamiliar staff	• Use facility protocol: Communicating with the Person with Dementia. • Reassess language use monthly for 3 months, then quarterly thereafter, to assure all favorite phrases and words are identified and well-known to staff.
Modify the environment to support losses.	Continuing activity needs	• Encourage participation in Vera's favorite activities: pet-resident interactions, walking in therapeutic gardens, plant care, cooking, visiting aviary, and telephone, and personal visits.
Provide on-going education, support, care and assistance with problem-solving to caregivers.		• Encourage participation in intergenerational programs as tolerated. • Assist Vera to alternate structured activities with "quiet time". • Review problems, issues, questions with DCNM during twice weekly visits (which will continue until Vera is adjusted). • Adjust care plans monthly for 3 months then quarterly thereafter.

Abbreviation: PAINAD, pain assessment in advanced dementia.

cares, cursing loudly at staff and other residents. She struck out repeatedly when pushed to "keep trying," hitting several staff. Pacing, general agitation, irritability, and exit-seeking behaviors increased, including a "close call" escape out the front door. An order for antipsychotic medication was obtained from the facility's medical director, and soon after, Vera was "sedate." The assistant nurse manager began arrangements for Vera's transfer to the facility's secure intermediate care unit where she could be "appropriately supervised" until other plans could be made. This "change in status" required notification of the DCNM who then demanded that a care conference be held.

Although the DCNM made every effort to explain Vera's behavior based on the PLST model, and offered alternative methods for her care, the assistant nurse manager and her staff remained adamant that Vera was a "threat" to others in the SNF and needed to be moved. Use of antipsychotic medications, however, made that argument difficult, because Vera was now docile. Instead, the DCNM requested that Vera be transferred to a different nursing facility, one that did not offer skilled care, but that was closer to her own home.

The facility she requested provided PT, OT, and dietician services by contract, not as part of their continuum of services. Relative to the SNF, it was considerably smaller but more specialized by having adopted "Eden Alternative™" care practices [25,26]. Like other "Edenized" programs, this facility strived to eliminate loneliness, boredom, and helplessness associated with aging and long-term care placement. The facility and its staff sought to redefine the care environment by incorporating animals, interactions with children, gardening, and an activity-focus to maximize resident participation and interaction with others.[6]

Given Vera's love of the outdoors, including plants and animals, the DCNM considered this facility the best alternative to assisted living or returning home—both of which seemed out of reach at the time. The facility was only 20 miles away from Vera's home town, which would allow more regular visits by neighbors and friends and use of adult day health services when that option became reasonable and placed Vera again under the care of her long-time family physician. Given the current circumstances, the DCNM worked diligently to get all parties involved to agree to the transfer. Once family members were reached and expressed support for the plan, Vera's family physician conceded that the "Edenized" facility might provide a superior alternative to the SNF. Refer to Table 4 to review the PLST care plan implemented at the new facility.

---

[6]The care concepts proposed by Thomas (1996) have been embraced by long-term facilities, their staffs, and state regulatory bodies alike (eg, state agencies in North Carolina and Missouri have adopted Eden concepts for use in long-term care facilities statewide). However, empirical evidence to support the model is limited. For more information on the model, visit the Eden website at http://www.edenalt.com/welcome.htm and search Pub Med http://www.ncbi.nlm.nih.gov/entrez/query.fcgi?db=PubMed to access recent literature (eg, see Bergman-Evans B, Beyond the basics. Effects of the Eden Alternative model on quality of life issues. J Gerontol Nurs 2004;30(6):27–34).

Edenized Facility Provides a More Homelike Setting

Entering the Eden Alternative™ facility, Vera was warmly welcomed by staff who introduced her to other residents and engaged her in activities that used her remaining abilities. As before, the DCNM worked in collaboration with staff to develop a personalized plan of care that followed the PLST model. An inservice program was provided to assure that staff were familiar with concepts previously used to promote function and comfort for Vera. Given the extensive overlap in Eden and PLST approaches to care, staff quickly grasped the ideas and implemented strategies with little difficulty. Antipsychotic medication was eliminated at the time of admission and an array of nonpharmacologic interventions, all consistent with her earlier patterns of living at home in the ALF, were reinstituted. Delirium-related confusion quickly resolved in the new care setting, and irritability and other behavioral symptoms subsided.

Within a short time, Vera returned to her typically amiable baseline behavior, as observed before Halloween. She told her family and visitors that she loved her new "condo," where she had lots of plants and new friends. Initially, she had some reservations about having companion animals in "her house,"; however, she was quickly adopted by one of the facility cats who allowed Vera to hold and cuddle him. Vera socialized and attended most activities with other residents and often entertained herself by watching birds in the aviary and walking in the therapeutic gardens, a secure outdoor area that was visible from her room's window. As before, she enjoyed assisting with meal preparation and other food-related activities in the facility. Of perhaps most importance, efforts to leave the facility and requests to "go home" subsided.

Margaret and Peter agreed that the DCNM had found an exemplary facility that met their mother's needs. The infusion of homelike activities, which were highly consistent with Vera's lifelong patterns of living, offered reassurance that their mother would be comfortable in the new setting. The staff were highly knowledgeable about dementia and were attentive to Vera's current and changing abilities. Given that Vera had adapted well to the novel new setting, Margaret and Peter agreed that Vera would remain at the facility for as long as possible.

SUMMARY

As the aging population continues to increase in the next decades, Alzheimer's disease and related dementias will become increasingly prevalent. Older adults with dementia are found in every setting imaginable today: living at home alone; living with family, friends, or hired caregivers; in adult day treatment programs; and living in assisted living facilities, group homes, foster care, residential facilities and nursing homes, including those with and without dementia-care units. As illustrated in the case vignette, the PLST model provides a useful approach for planning and evaluating care across settings. The model is understood easily by nonprofessional caregivers, allows flexibility to modify the plan of care based on the person's changing needs, and can be applied by knowledgeable nurses with diverse specialty backgrounds.

References
[1] IPA. Behavioral and psychological symptoms of dementia (BPSD). Skogie (IL): International Psychogeriatric Association; 2003.
[2] Hall GR, Buckwalter KC. Progressively lowered stress threshold: a conceptual model for care of adults with Alzheimer's disease. Arch Psychiatr Nurs 1987;1(6):399–406.
[3] Smith M, Gerdner L, Hall GR, et al. History, development, and future of the Progressively Lowered Stress Threshold: a conceptual model for dementia care. J Am Geriatr Soc 2004;52(10):1755–60.
[4] Hall GR, Buckwalter KC, Stolley JM, et al. Standardized care plan: managing Alzheimer's patients at home. J Gerontol Nurs 1995;21(1):37–49.
[5] Wolanin M, Phillips L. Confusion: prevention and care. St. Louis (MO): Mosby; 1981.
[6] Lazarus R. Psychological stress and coping. New York: McGraw-Hill; 1966.
[7] Verwoerdt A. Anxiety, dissociative and personality disorders in the elderly. In: Busse E, Blazer D, editors. Handbook of geriatric psychiatry. New York: Van Nostrand Reinhold; 1980. p. 368–89.
[8] Rogers CR. Client-centered therapy: its current practice, implications, and theory. Boston: Houghton Mifflin; 1951.
[9] Nahemow L. The ecological theory of aging: Powel Lawton's legacy. In: Rubinstine RL, Moss M, Keban MH, editors. The many dimensions of aging. New York: Springer Publishing; 2000. p. 22–40.
[10] Gerdner LA, Hall GR, Buckwalter KC. Caregiver training for people with Alzheimer's based on a stress threshold model. Image J Nurs Sch 1996;28(3):241–6.
[11] Buckwalter K, Smith M, Mitchell S. When you forget that you forgot: recognizing and managing Alzheimer's type dementia. In: Smith M, Buckwalter K, Mitchell S, editors. The geriatric mental health training series. New York: Springer Publishing Company; 1993.
[12] Hall GR, Buckwalter KC. Whole disease care planning: fitting the program to the client with Alzheimer's disease. J Gerontol Nurs 1991;17(3):38–41.
[13] Hall GR, Gerdner L, Zwygart-Stauffacher M, et al. Principles of nonpharmocological management: Caring for people with Alzheimer's disease using a conceptual model. Psychiatr Ann 1995;25(7):432–40.
[14] Hall GR. Care of the patient with Alzheimer's disease living at home. Nurs Clin North Am 1988;23(1):31–46.
[15] Swanson EA, Maas ML, Buckwalter KC. Alzheimer's residents' cognitive and functional measures: Special and traditional care unit comparison. Clin Nurs Res 1994;3(1): 27–41.
[16] Hall GR, Kirschling MV, Todd S. Sheltered freedom: the creation of a special care Alzheimer's unit in an intermediate level facility. Geriatr Nurs (Minneap) 1986;7(3):56–63.
[17] Stolley JM, Hall GR, Collins J, et al. Managing the care of patients with irreversible dementia during hospitalization for comorbidities. Nurs Clin North Am 1993;28(4):767–82.
[18] Hall GR, Specht J, Bossen A, et al. Evaluating persons with dementia who live alone: a quick assessment for knowing when to intervene. Manuscript submitted for publication; 2005.
[19] Gerdner L. Individualized music intervention protocol. J Gerontol Nurs 1999;25(10): 10–6.
[20] Warden V, Hurley A, Volicer L. Development and psychometric evaluation of the PAINAD (Pain Assessment in Advanced Dementia) scale. J Am Med Dir Assoc 2003;4(1):9–15.
[21] Folstein MF, Folstein SE, McHugh PR. "Mini-Mental State"—a practical method for grading the cognitive state of patients for the clinician. J Psychiatr Res 1975;12:189–98.
[22] Inouye SK, Van Dyke DC, Alessi CA, et al. Clarifying confusion: the confusion assessment method. A new approach for detection of delirium. Ann Intern Med 1990;113(2):941–8.
[23] Hall GR. Outside the box: restraint alternatives that work in acute care. Available at: http://www.centeronaging.uiowa.edu/pubs/Newest%20Versions%20-%20pdf%20format/Outside%20the%20Box.pdf; 2005. Accessed June 25, 2005.

[24] Cohen-Mansfield J. Instruction Manual for the Cohen-Mansfield Agitation Inventory (CMAI). Rockville (MD): Research Institute of the Hebrew Home of Greater Washington; 1991.
[25] Thomas W. Life worth living. Acton (MA): VanderWyk & Burnham; 1996.
[26] Thomas W, Stermer M. Eden Alternative Principles hold promise for the future of long-term care. Balance 1999;3(4):14–7.

Nurs Clin N Am 41 (2006) 83–93

NURSING CLINICS
OF NORTH AMERICA

Alzheimer's Disease: Issues and Challenges in Primary Care

Valerie T. Cotter, MSN, CRNP, FAANP

School of Nursing, 420 Guardian Drive, University of Pennsylvania, Philadelphia, PA 19104, USA

A 73-year-old woman presents for an initial visit at a primary care office and is accompanied by her daughter. The daughter is concerned that her mother could not recall the names of some cousins at a recent family reunion and thinks that she is slightly less engaged in life than before. The patient says, "I'm no worse than someone else my age." What advice would you offer her and the family regarding possible cognitive decline?

THE CLINICAL DILEMMA IN PRIMARY CARE

Approximately 4.5 million Americans are affected by Alzheimer's disease (AD), and the prevalence is predicted to increase to 13.2 million by 2050 [1]. Advancing age is the single greatest risk factor to develop AD. The number of newly diagnosed individuals with AD, as shown in Fig. 1, increases from about 0.17% at 65 years of age to 3% at 85 years of age, with a dramatic increase to 8% per year after age 85 [2]. These United States prevalence and incidence figures are consistent with similar cross-cultural studies in Europe and Japan. With the demographic shift to an aging population, it is imperative for nurses working in primary care to be knowledgeable about care of individuals who have AD.

The challenge in primary care practice is identifying persons with symptoms of AD who often have limited capacity to recognize their own symptoms and attribute cognitive decline to chronic illness or aging. Brief office visit communications without an informant, such as a spouse or adult child rarely uncover mild stage AD. Clinicians in primary care fail to screen older adults for AD on a routine basis because of insufficient time, inadequate reimbursement for services, and uncertainty about the value of an early diagnosis. Although current pharmacologic and behavioral interventions and patient education do not prevent eventual disease progression, they arguably lead to improvements in understanding, self-efficacy, and quality of life for the patient and family.

E-mail address: cottervt@nursing.upenn.edu

0029-6465/06/$ – see front matter
doi:10.1016/j.cnur.2005.09.005 nursing.theclinics.com

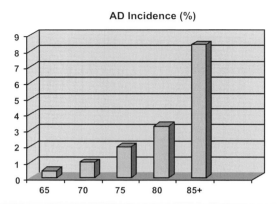

Fig 1. Age specific incidence rates of AD.

SCREENING IN PRIMARY CARE PRACTICE

In a traditional model of secondary preventive services, detection of early stage disease and treatment efficacy is fundamental in determining the clinical value of a screening test. It fails to take into account the burden of mistaking the earliest symptoms for another condition or not knowing the diagnosis to adequately plan for the future. Apparent cognitive or functional decline always is relevant clinically, regardless of how mild the symptoms may be. Informing patients and their family members that periodic screening for AD, the most common neurodegenerative dementia is a worthwhile, low-cost strategy for beneficial quality-of-life effects. For example, when a spouse understands that apathetic symptoms are not an intentional, indifferent attitude but a common behavioral manifestation in AD, it can lead to improved communication between the patient and spouse. Another argument for early diagnosis is that it makes it possible for the person with AD to participate in future planning on important issues, such as financial, legal, and living arrangements, and helps the family seek out community resources to reduce the stress of caregiving.

Because the earliest symptoms of AD include memory loss for recent events and impairment in another cognitive domain (language, executive function, visuo-spatial skills, calculation abilities, attention, and judgment) that is significant to impair everyday functioning, the screening instruments should test these areas. Several reliable and valid instruments are available for screening and serial evaluations in the primary care setting. An evaluation that includes brief cognitive testing with the patient and collecting a history of cognitive and functional performance from an informant is most effective [3,4].

These assessments can be administered by trained nurses working in a primary care community health center or office-based practice as part of an annual or new patient visit. In this method, patients who are found to have cognitive or functional impairments suggestive of AD are evaluated more extensively at a subsequent visit or referred to a neurologist or dementia specialist. Those patients already identified with AD are followed with serial cognitive and functional assessments to assess progression and implement supportive strategies for the patient and family.

BRIEF COGNITIVE TESTS

The Mini-Mental State Exam (MMSE) tests memory, orientation, and attention, as well as ability to name, follow verbal and written instructions, write a sentence, and copy an intersecting polygon [5]. A score of 24 or above, out of a maximum score of 30 is considered normal, though age and education influences the result. Generally, increased age and lower education level attainment result in lower MMSE scores. In a large-scale population study, the median MMSE score in a 75-year-old person varied greatly depending upon education level: 0 to 4 years of education was 21 (SD 2.1); 9 to 12 years of education was 27 (SD 1.5), and college experience or degree was 28 (SD 1.6) [6].

The Mini-Cog, a briefer cognitive screen combining a three-item recall and clock drawing, shown in Fig. 2, performs as well or better than the MMSE [7]. When using the MMSE cutoff score of 24, the Mini-Cog has higher sensitivity (76%) than the MMSE (71%) but lower specificity (89% versus 94%). When the MMSE cutoff is raised to 25, the Mini-Cog and MMSE have similar sensitivity and specificity for identifying dementia, uninfluenced by age or education.

FUNCTIONAL AND BEHAVIORAL ASSESSMENT

Functional and behavioral symptoms are not correlated necessarily with cognitive symptoms in AD; therefore, detailed functional and behavioral assessments should be included as part of an initial or serial cognitive assessment. Functional impairment in advanced activities of daily living (AADLs), such as work, hobbies, or social activities and instrumental activities of daily living (IADLs), such as shopping, household maintenance, money management, driving, cooking, laundry, and use of the telephone are defining features in early stage AD. As the disease progresses into moderate and late stages, basic activities of daily living (ADLs), including bathing, dressing, grooming, continence, ambulation, and eating are affected. A functional assessment instrument completed by a family member or someone who knows the patient helps to assess whether there is significant functional impairment to diagnose AD or define the stage of AD.

The 11-item Dementia Severity Rating Scale (DSRS), an informant-based scale increases as the patients' disease severity increases and can help differentiate AD from normal cognitive function: less than 4 in normal cognition; 7 to 10 in mild cognitive impairment; 11 to 21 in mild stage AD; 22 to 32 in moderate stage AD; and 33 to 47 in severe stage AD [8]. The informant should be instructed to complete each item based on cognitive dysfunction not a physical impairment. For example, in a person who has limited mobility and inability to drive or take public transportation related to osteoarthritis more than AD, the mobility/walking item is likely to be in the lower range.

DATE_____ PT INIITIALS _____ #_____ AGE____ GENDER M F CLINIC NAME_____ PROVIDER_____ TESTED BY_____

MINI-COG ™

1) GET THE PATIENT'S ATTENTION, THEN SAY: "I am going to say three words that I want you to remember. The words are
   Banana   Sunrise   Chair.
   Please say them for me now." (Give the patient 3 tries to repeat the words. If unable after 3 tries, go to next item.)
   (Fold this page back at the TWO dotted lines BELOW to make a blank space and cover the memory words. Hand the patient a pencil/pen).
2) SAY ALL THE FOLLOWING PHRASES IN THE ORDER INDICATED: "Please draw a clock in the space below. Start by drawing a large
   circle." (When this is done, say) "Put all the numbers in the circle." (When done, say) "**Now set the hands to show 11:10 (10 past 11).**"

---

3) SAY: "What were the three words I asked you to remember?"

_____   _____   _____   (Score 1 point for each) 3-Item Recall Score   [ ]

Score the clock (see other side for instructions):   Normal clock   2 points   Clock Score   [ ]
                                                      Abnormal clock 0 points

Total Score = 3-item recall plus clock score   [ ]   *0, 1, or 2 possible impairment; 3, 4, or 5 suggests no impairment*

CLOCK SCORING

NORMAL CLOCK

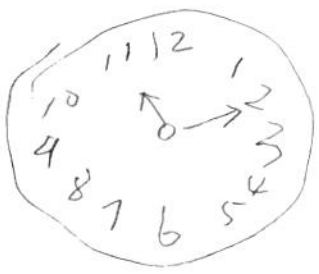

A NORMAL CLOCK HAS ALL OF THE FOLLOWING ELEMENTS:
All numbers 1-12, each only once, are present in the correct order and direction (clockwise).
Two hands are present, one pointing to 11 and one pointing to 2.

ANY CLOCK MISSING EITHER OF THESE ELEMENTS IS SCORED ABNORMAL. REFUSAL TO DRAW A CLOCK IS SCORED ABNORMAL.

SOME EXAMPLES OF ABNORMAL CLOCKS (THERE ARE MANY OTHER KINDS)

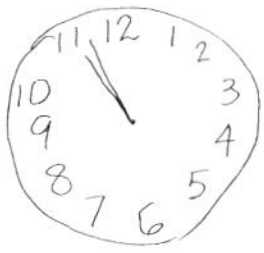

Abnormal Hands 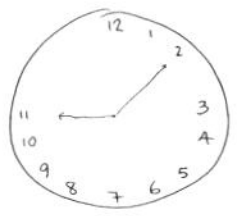   Abnormal Spacing 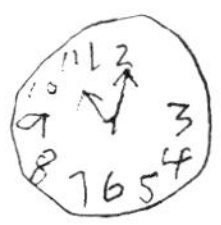   Abnormal Spacing/Numbers

Fig 2. Mini-Cog.

Mental and behavioral symptoms, such as delusions, visual hallucinations, sleep disturbances, apathy, and psychomotor restlessness, are prevalent in AD and associated with increasing disease severity. In a study of community-dwelling elders with dementia and no behavioral symptoms, 69% developed at least one mental or behavioral symptom (delusions 28%, apathy 21%, and wandering/pacing behaviors 21%) within 18 months [9]. Behavioral symptoms are the one patient characteristic that predicts caregiver depression and earlier nursing home placement [10].

A neurobiologic, extrinsic, and environmental basis for their origin exists, which is why a broad-based approach to patient management is most effective. In primary care settings, the nurse should include routine assessments of behavior in AD as one takes a blood pressure reading in a patient who has hypertension. This assessment could be easily incorporated into the visit by using a behavioral checklist with the family when in the waiting room or during the initial encounter with the patient. A helpful tool in regards to persistent behavioral symptoms is a take-home log or diary to determine more details of the specific symptoms, the timing of their occurrence, and the response to interventions. Greater involvement between the nurse and the caregiver results in better understanding of the relationship among AD symptoms and disease progression and emphasizes a more flexible approach to problem solving and management.

STAGING AD

Disease severity is categorized commonly into mild, moderate, and severe stages. Mild stage AD is the longest, typically occurring up to 4 years, moderate stage occurring 2 to 3 years, and severe stage occurring 1 to 3 years. It is clinically useful to characterize severe stage disease further into profound and terminal stages to help predict the time when hospice services will benefit the patient and family.

Stage-defined characteristics include cognition, behavior, and functional abilities, as shown in Table 1. Understanding the various stages of AD is necessary when considering pharmacologic and behavioral interventions for the patient, and caregiver educational and supportive approaches (Table 2). The average duration of AD from diagnosis to death is 8 years, though median survival of a person diagnosed at age 65 is 9 years and 3 years in a person diagnosed at 90 years [11].

FAMILY CAREGIVERS

Most people who have AD are cared for at home by family or friends spending an average of 17.6 hours per week giving care [12]. The caregiver, often a daughter or daughter-in-law, has a critical role in maintaining the patient's overall quality of life and is at risk themselves for psychiatric and physical morbidity from the stresses of caregiving [10]. Several studies report improved patient and caregiver outcomes with interventions directed at the caregiver. A randomized controlled trial of spouse caregivers of patients with mild to moderate stage AD involving a 4 month program of weekly support groups, 4–6 counseling sessions to provide emotional support, education about AD and available resources, and management of behavioral symptoms, and continuous phone availability of counselors delayed nursing home placement one-year

Table 1
Stages of dementia

	Mild	Moderate	Severe	Profound	Terminal
Function	• IADL independent or decreased ability with complex tasks • ADL independent	• IADL dependent or assistance needed • ADL independent or reminders, assistance needed	• IADL dependent • ADL dependent (incontinent, able to feed self, still ambulatory)	• IADL dependent • ADL dependent (loss of ambulation, feeds with assistance)	• Inability to walk or sit up without assistance • Inability to smile or hold head up • >10% body weight loss, pressure ulcers >stage 2, UTI, aspiration pneumonia • Few words spoken
Cognition	• Difficulty learning new information, memory loss interferes with everyday functions • Difficulty with time relationships • Mild word-finding difficulty • Able to carry on social conversation • Mild judgment impairment	• Substantial memory loss, disoriented in time, often to place • Conversation disorganized, rambling • Judgment impaired • Decreased attention span	• Oriented to person only • Only fragments of memory remain • Severe language impairment • Inconsistent recognition of familiar people • Short attention span	• Speaks < 6 words • Consistent difficulty recognizing familiar people	

Behavior	• Mild personality changes • Less engaged in relationships • Appears normal	• May have psychotic, wandering, elopement, agitated verbal or physical symptoms • Sleep disturbance • Appears well enough to be taken to functions outside home	• Emotional lability • Restlessness • Inability to focus on tasks • Appears too ill to be taken to functions outside home	• Repetitive vocalizations, calling out • More passive	• Passive
Cognitive scores	• MMSE ≥ 19	• MMSE 12–19	• MMSE 6–11	• MMSE < 6	• Not testable

Abbreviations: ADL, activities of daily living; IADL, instrumental activities of daily living; MMSE, Mini-Mental State Exam; UTI, urinary tract infection.

Adapted from Cotter VT. Forgetfulness. In: Goolsby MJ, editor. Nurse practitioner secrets. Philadelphia: Hanley & Belfus; 2002. p. 68.

Table 2
Stage-based nursing interventions for patient-caregiver dyad

	Mild	Moderate	Severe	Profound	Terminal
Patient	• Information about AD, treatment • ChEI • Driving evaluation • Discussion re-interdependence on CG and others (AADL, IADL) • Discussion with CG re-preferences for future health care, financial and legal needs • Advance directive, power of attorney • Activities to promote well-being (peer support, volunteer work)	• Safe return identification as long as patient is ambulatory • ChEI; memantine • Supportive nonverbal communication with CG • Structured environment • Adult day program 2–3 times weekly • 24-hour supervision	• ChEI; memantine • Adult day program 2–3 times weekly • 24-hour assistance • Adequate nutrition, hydration, mobility, pain and behavior management	• Life-sustaining approaches without artificial nutrition, hydration • 24-hour assistance • Conservative treatment of co-morbid conditions • Reduce complications from falls, infection, dysphagia, pressure ulcers	• Referral to hospice program • 24-hour assistance • Comfort care • Life-sustaining approaches without artificial nutrition, hydration
Caregiver	• Information about AD, treatment, community resources • Peer support • Learn CG role	• Share CG tasks with others • Regular respite • Peer support • Education re-communication, behavioral strategies • Discussion re-long term care at home and in a facility	• Education re-palliative care symptom management (nutrition, hydration, mobility, pain, behavior), ADL care, prevention of hospitalization • Peer support	• Bereavement services • Regular respite • Peer support	• Bereavement services, support for future plans • Peer support

Abbreviations: CG, caregiver; ChEI, cholinesterase inhibitor.

longer [13]. This intervention has also been shown to reduce caregiver depression symptoms within the first year and have longer lasting results beyond 3 years [14,15]. The implications of these findings for nursing are clear: counseling, education, and support for the caregiver have important outcomes for the patient and family and should be incorporated within primary care practice by nurses.

PHARMACOLOGIC INTERVENTIONS

At each stage of AD, nurses should consider the clinical benefits and adverse effects of pharmacologic interventions in the care of the patient. Because patients rely on a caregiver to administer medications and monitor response, nurses need to develop good communication patterns with the caregiver and have useful educational materials on hand to distribute at a primary care visit or to recommend for outside readings and resources. Web-based literature and sites, such as the Alzheimer's Association (www.alz.org) [16] and Alzheimer's Disease Education and Referral Center (www.alzheimers.org) [17], and email communication can be very effective and time efficient methods of communication and education with many caregivers.

In mild to moderate stage, cholinesterase inhibitors (ChEIs) are thought to increase the availability of acetylcholine at receptor sites in the neocortex and hippocampus and improve the symptoms of cognition, mood and behavior. Second generation ChEIs, donepezil hydrochloride, galantamine hydrobromide, and rivastigmine are approved by the Federal Food and Drug Administration in mild to moderate AD. Multiple studies have shown modest clinical benefits in the earlier stages; however, little evidence exists to support continued use into advanced stages [18–21]. Common adverse effects, such as nausea, vomiting, diarrhea, anorexia, and bradycardia, are often transient when the drug is initiated and occur at higher doses.

Overstimulation of the neurotransmitter glutamate may result in neuronal calcium overload and cell damage and ultimately stimulate N-methyl-D-aspartate (NMDA) receptors. Memantine, a NMDA antagonist studied in moderate to severe stage patients not taking a ChEI, showed more positive effects on the cognitive and functional symptoms, as compared with the placebo group in a 28-week trial [22]. More recently, a randomized controlled 24-week trial of memantine and stable doses of donepezil in moderate to severe stage patients (MMSE 5-14) demonstrated modest outcomes on cognitive, functional, and behavioral outcomes [23]. The most frequent side effects of memantine include agitation, insomnia, and diarrhea.

SUMMARY

As the number of individuals who have AD continues to increase, nurses become the frontline providers in primary care settings. The challenge is to recognize early symptoms and intervene by preparing the person who has AD and caregivers through the progression of the disease. By counseling, educating, and supporting the caregiver and maximizing the patient's quality of life through pharmacologic and behavioral interventions, nurses can provide a much-needed broad-based approach to their care.

References

[1] Hebert LE, Scherr PA, Bienias JL, et al. Alzheimer disease in the US population: prevalence estimates using the 2000 census. Arch Neurol 2003;60:1119–22.

[2] Brookmeyer R, Gray S, Kawas C. Projections of Alzheimer's disease in the United States and the public health impact of delaying disease onset. Am J Public Health 1998;88(9): 1337–42.

[3] Cotter VT, Clark CM, Karlawish JHT. Cognitive function assessment in individuals at risk for Alzheimer's disease. JAANP 2003;15(2):79–86.

[4] Tierney MC, Herrmann N, Geslani DM, et al. Contribution of informant and patient ratings to the accuracy of the Mini-Mental State Examination in predicting probable Alzheimer's disease. JAGS 2003;51:813–8.

[5] Folstein MF, Folstein SE, McHugh PR. Mini-Mental State: a practical method for grading the cognitive state of patients for the clinician. J Psychiat Res 1975;12(3):189–98.

[6] Crum RM, Anthony JC, Bassett SS, et al. Population-based norms for the Mini-Mental State Examination by age and educational level. JAMA 1993;269(18):2386–91.

[7] Borson S, Scanlan JM, Chen P, et al. The Mini-Cog as a screen for dementia: validation in a population-based sample. JAGS 2003;51(10):1451–4.

[8] Clark CM, Ewbank DC. Performance of the Dementia Severity Rating Scale: a caregiver questionnaire for rating severity in Alzheimer disease. Alzheimer Dis Assoc Disord 1996;10:31–9.

[9] Steinberg M, Sheppard JM, Tschanz JT, et al. The incidence of mental and behavioral disturbances in dementia: the CACHE County study. J Neuropsychiatry Clin Neurosci 2003;15:340–5.

[10] Schulz R, O'Brien AT, Bookwala J, et al. Psychiatric and physical morbidity effects of dementia caregiving: prevalence, correlates, and causes. Gerontologist 1995;15(5): 771–91.

[11] Brookmeyer R, Corrada MM, Curriero FC, et al. Survival following a diagnosis of Alzheimer's disease. Arch Neurol 2002;59:1764–7.

[12] Alzheimer's Association and the National Alliance for Caregiving. Who cares? Washington, DC: Alzheimer's Association; 1999. p. 1–15.

[13] Mittelman MS, Ferris SH, Shulman E, et al. A family intervention to delay nursing home placement of patients with Alzheimer disease. JAMA 1996;276(21):1725–31.

[14] Mittelman MS, Ferris SH, Shulman E, et al. A comprehensive support program: Effect on depression in spouse-caregivers of AD patients. Gerontologist 1995;35:792–802.

[15] Mittelman MS, Roth DL, Coon DW, et al. Sustained benefit of supportive intervention for depressive symptoms in caregivers of patients with Alzheimer's disease. Am J Psychiatry 2004;161(5):850–6.

[16] Alzheimer's Association. Available at: http://www.alz.org. Accessed July 10, 2005.

[17] Alzheimer's Disease Education and Referral Center. Available at: http://www.alzheimers. org. Accessed July 10, 2005.

[18] Raskind MA, Peskind ER, Wessel T, et al for the Galantamine Study Group. Galantamine in AD: a 6-month randomized, placebo-controlled trial with a 6-month extension. Neurology 2000;54:2261–8.

[19] Rogers SL, Farlow MR, Doody RS, et al for the Donepezil Study Group. A 24-week, double-blind, placebo-controlled trial of donepezil in patients with Alzheimer's disease. Neurology 1998;50:136–45.

[20] Grossberg G, Irwin P, Satlin A, et al. Rivastigmine in Alzheimer's disease: efficacy over two years. Am J Geriatr Psychiatry 2004;12:420–31.
[21] Grutzendler J, Morris JC. Cholinesterase inhibitors for Alzheimer's disease. Drugs 2001;61(1):41–52.
[22] Reisberg B, Doody R, Stoffler A, et al, for the Memantine Study Group. Memantine in moderate-to-severe Alzheimer's disease. N Engl J Med 2003;348(14):1333–41.
[23] Tariot PN, Farlow MR, Grossberg GT, et al. Memantine treatment in patients with moderate to severe Alzheimer's disease already receiving donepezil. JAMA 2004;291:317–24.

Nurs Clin N Am 41 (2006) 95–104

NURSING CLINICS
OF NORTH AMERICA

Measuring the Quality of Nursing Care to Alzheimer's Patients

Ivo L. Abraham, PhD, RN, CS, FAAN[a,b,c,d,e,*],
Karen M. MacDonald, PhD, RN[a],
Deborah M. Nadzam, PhD, RN, FAAN[f,g]

[a]Matrix45, 620 Frays Ridge Road, Earlysville, VA 22936, USA
[b]Center for Health Outcomes and Policy Research, School of Nursing & Leonard Davis Institute of Health Economics, Wharton School of Business, University of Pennsylvania, Philadelphia, PA, USA
[c]College of Nursing, University of Arizona, Tucson, AZ, USA
[d]School of Nursing, New York University, New York, NY, USA
[e]School of Nursing, University of Virginia, Charlottesville, VA, USA
[f]Institute for Healthcare Quality, The Cleveland Clinic Health System, Cleveland, OH, USA
[g]Frances Payne Bolton School of Nursing, Case Western Reserve University, Cleveland, OH, USA

F acilities that provide care to Alzheimer's disease patients (adult day care centers, assisted living facilities, skilled nursing facilities, and other facilities) are under unrelenting pressure to document the quality of nursing care they provide to various stakeholders: patients, families, managers, communities, payers, regulators, and accreditors. Unfortunately, little consensus exists nor is guidance given as to *how* to measure the quality of nursing care. True, regulations and standards exist but are seldom translated into systematic outcome measures that assist nurses and facilities to measure, report, and manage the quality of care they provide to residents in general and Alzheimer's patients in particular. This article offers practical advice on conceptualizing quality of nursing care to Alzheimer's patients and the selection of outcome measures to collect, analyze, use, and report quality of nursing care data. This article does not recommend specific measures but encourages you to take the important earlier step: knowing what constitutes good and poor measures and how to select them in function of a quality management program.

Is it possible to measure the quality of nursing care provided to Alzheimer's patients? Can direct indicators of quality be identified (eg, "this indicator shows quality nursing care is being provided")? Or do indirect indicators have to be relied on (eg, "if indicator 'x' drops, can it be reasonably inferred an improvement in the quality of nursing care is occurring?")? What factors may influence

*Matrix45, 620 Frays Ridge Road, Earlysville, VA 22936, USA. *E-mail address*: iabraham@matrix45.com (I.L. Abraham).

0029-6465/06/$ – see front matter
doi:10.1016/j.cnur.2005.09.002

desired quality outcomes? How can evaluation programs be designed that enable quality to be measured without adding significant burden and taking time away from direct patient care? How "scientific" should quality monitoring be? Should it be as objective and rigorous as a research study? Should the outcomes of care be benchmarked to established guidelines or standards of nursing care for geriatric patients and those with Alzheimer's disease in particular?

It would be ideal if this article could provide answers to all of these questions; however, no consensus exists, nor may it ever, as to how to measure quality of nursing care in general and to Alzheimer's patients in particular. Furthermore, if *the* model of quality measurement existed, would it be relevant to all possible clinical sites? Implementable without burdensome procedures and resource demands? Sufficiently operational to enable quality improvement? This article provides guidance in the selection, development, and use of outcome measures to monitor quality of care. Following a definition of quality, several challenges in the measurement of quality are identified. The concept of outcome measures is then introduced and practical advice on how to measure performance is offered. The article concludes with a review of common problems in the measurement of outcomes of nursing care in general, to geriatric patients, and to Alzheimer's patients.

MANAGING QUALITY OF NURSING CARE

A Process, Not a State

The Institute of Medicine (IOM) [1] defines quality of care as the degree to which health services for individuals and populations increase the likelihood of desired health outcomes and are consistent with current professional knowledge. Interestingly, this definition does *not* tell us what quality is but what quality should achieve. The definition does *not* say that quality exists if certain conditions are met but instead puts the emphasis on the likelihood of achieving desired levels of care. Quality of nursing care is not a matter of reaching something (eg, "we've got it!") but rather the challenge, over and over, of improving the odds of reaching the desired level of outcomes (eg, "where are we and where do we go from here?"). Thus, the definition implies the cyclic and longitudinal nature of quality: what we achieve today must guide us to what to do tomorrow—better and better, over and over. The IOM definition also stresses the framework within which to conceptualize quality: knowledge. The best knowledge to have is research evidence – preferably from randomized clinical trials or experimental studies yet without ignoring the relevance of less rigorous studies (eg, nonrandomized studies, epidemiologic investigations, descriptive studies, even case studies). Realistically, in (geriatric) nursing limited evidence is available to guide our care; therefore, professional consensus among clinical and research experts is a critical factor in determining quality. The knowledge element occurs at three levels: (1) to achieve quality, it is necessary to know *what to do* (knowledge about *best practice*); (2) it is necessary to know *how to do it* (knowledge about *best skills*); and (3) it is necessary to know *what outcomes to achieve* (knowledge about *best outcomes*). The IOM definition contains several other important elements. "Health services" focus the definition on care itself. The definition implies a challenge to health care organizations small and large: organize yourself in such a way that knowledge-based care is provided and that its effects can be measured.

This point brings us to the "outcomes" element of the definition. Quality is not an attribute (eg, "my skilled nursing facility is in the top five percent in the state") but an ability (as in: "only 'x' percent of my Alzheimer's patients exhibit agitation during meals; however, playing soothing music during meals reduces that by 'y' percent"). In the IOM definition, "degree" implies that quality occurs on a continuum from low to high, from unacceptable to excellent. Degree also implies quantification—trying to put a number to it. Though it helps to talk to colleagues about, say, unacceptable, poor, average, good, or excellent nursing care to Alzheimer's patients, these terms should be anchored by a measurement system that enables interpretation of what, for instance, poor nursing care is by providing a range of numbers that correspond to "poor." In turn, these numbers provide a reference point for improving care to the level of average: measure the care again, look whether the numbers have improved, and then check whether these numbers fall within the range of numbers defined as "average." Likewise, if a worsening of scores occurs, it can be inferred that the care has gone from "good" to "average."

The IOM definition's reference to "individuals and populations" underscores that quality of care is reflected in the outcomes of *one* patient and in the outcomes of a *set* of patients. The definition focuses our attention on providing quality nursing care to individuals with Alzheimer's disease while aiming to raise the level of care that is provided to populations of Alzheimer's patients. In summary, the IOM definition forces thinking about quality in relative and dynamic terms rather than in absolute and static terms. Quality of nursing care to Alzheimer's patients is not a state of being but a process of becoming. This quality is and should be measurable, and for this outcome measures are necessary, quantitative tools that provide an indication of performance in relation to a specified process or outcome.

In the Eye of the Beholder

If the IOM definition is so helpful, why is there such divergence in operationalizing quality of care and designing quality management programs in health care in general, in nursing, and in the care of Alzheimer's patients? Quality of nursing is in the eye of the beholder. For instance, nurses wonder whether they, as individual practitioners, provide good care and how they can become better at what they do. They may also wonder whether they work for a good organization: one that consistently provides good care to all its patients and challenges itself to find new and better ways of serving their patients. Facilities worry about the relationship with their patients and, certainly in the case of Alzheimer's care, the patients' families. Administrators worry about payment, reimbursement, accreditation, and contracting. Purchasers and payers of health care try to find ways of balancing quality and cost. Regulators and accreditors want assurances that safe care is being provided to Alzheimer's patients. For them, the issue is not one of top quality but rather of basic and necessary quality. Lastly, Alzheimer's patients and especially their families want assurances. They want the barriers to care lowered. They expect care to be safe—especially considering the vulnerability of the patient population. They hope that the care will make them better; or, at least, that suffering will be minimized.

Where do these divergent views on quality of care come from? They go back to the "process ('becoming') versus state ('being')" issue. Quality improvement is a process of attaining ever better levels of care paralleled with advances in knowledge and technology. It strives toward increasing the likelihood that certain outcomes will be achieved. This "becoming" is the professional responsibility of those who provide care to Alzheimer's patients—nurses, managers, and their organizations.

Measuring Quality of Care

Challenges

Schyve and Nadzam [2] identify numerous challenges to measuring quality of care, several of which apply to nursing care provided to Alzheimer's patients (Box 1).

Addressing the Challenges

These challenges are not insurmountable; however, making a commitment to quality nursing care entails a commitment to putting the processes and systems in place to measure quality through outcome measures and to report quality of care results. Once you decide to pursue excellence (ie, quality), you must accept measurement and reporting and overcome the various challenges. Examine

---

Box 1: Challenges

1. *Stakeholders.* Considering that quality of care is in the eye of the beholder, measurement and analysis methods must generate information about quality of care that meets the needs of different stakeholders. The results must be communicated in ways that are useful to each of the stakeholder groups.

2. *Measurement tools.* Good and generally accepted tools for measuring quality must be available. Notwithstanding their different needs, stakeholder groups must come together in their conceptualization of quality nursing care to Alzheimer's patients so that relevant measures can be identified and standardized. A common language of measurement must be developed, grounded in a shared perspective on quality that is cohesive across yet also meets the divergent needs of various stakeholder groups.

3. *Data collection.* Once the measurement systems are in place, data must be collected. This translates into resource demands and logistic issues as to who is to report, record, collect, and manage data.

4. *Data analysis.* Data must be analyzed in statistically appropriate ways. This analysis is not just a matter of using the right statistical methods. More importantly, user groups must agree on a framework for analyzing and interpreting quality of care data.

how this can be done in your clinical setting as you try to improve the quality of care to Alzheimer's patients. McGlynn and Asch [3] offer several strategies (Box 2).

In summary, the success of a quality management program in long-term care hinges on the decision of what to measure. Good outcome measures must be objective, data collection must be easy and minimally burdensome, statistical analysis must be girded by principles and placed within a framework, and communication of results must be targeted toward different user groups.

Conceivably, an attempt could be made to measure every possible aspect of our care, but realistically this is impossible. Instead, establish priorities by asking yourself: based on our clinical expertise, what is critical for us to know? what aspects of our care is high risk? what parts of our care are problem-prone, either because we have experienced difficulties in the past or we can anticipate problems caused by lack of knowledge or resources? what clinical indicators are of interest to other user groups: patients, families, the general public, management, payers, accreditors, and practitioners? Throughout this prioritization process, keep the bigger picture in mind, and continue to ask yourself what questions you are trying to answer and for whom.

Box 2: Addressing the challenges

1. *Common measurement platform.* The various user groups must balance competing perspectives. This balance is a process of give and take. Propose highly clinical measures to assist nurses, but also provide more general data for use by administrators.

2. *Accountability framework.* Committing to quality care implies that you assume several responsibilities and are willing to be held accountable for each of them: (a) providing the best possible care to Alzheimer's patients, (b) examining your own clinical knowledge and practice, (c) seeking ways to improve it, (d) agreeing to the evaluation of your practice, and (e) responding to needs for improvement.

3. *Objectivity in the evaluation of quality.* This challenge requires adopting explicit criteria for judging performance and building the evaluation process on these criteria. You, your colleagues, and your managers need to reach consensus on how performances are measured and what is considered "excellent" (and "good," "average," and so forth) performance.

4. *Routine reporting.* Once these indicators have been identified, select a subset of indicators for routine reporting that give a reliable snapshot of your care and your team's care to Alzheimer's patients.

5. *Separate quality and finance.* To avoid money driving quality of care or lack of money driving down quality of care, it is critical to minimize the use of clinical indicators for financial or nonfinancial (risk management, accreditation, and so forth) purposes. Should you be cost conscious? Yes, but cost should not influence your clinical judgment as to what is best for your patients.

MEASURING PERFORMANCE

Once you have decided what to measure, you must decide how to measure performance. Two possibilities are available: appropriate measures already exist or you face the task of developing a new outcome measure. Either way, numerous requirements of good outcome measures that you will need to apply to the decision process.

What Are Good Outcome Measures?

The question "is this a good measure?" can be answered in two ways. First, you must decide if the measure is of potential use to you and your organization in the day-to-day care of Alzheimer's patients. Once you've determined the usefulness of the measure, you should review its characteristics to determine if it is a good outcome measure in general (eg, well defined, tested, and so forth).

Usefulness

The process of selecting an outcome measure begins with two sets of questions about its usefulness.

Usefulness of the Measure

What do I need to know? What is the purpose of a given outcome measure? Do need and purpose match? If you cannot get to a "reasonable yes" on this first set of questions, the outcome measure you are reviewing may not meet your objectives. By "reasonable yes" we mean that your assessment of the match between your need and the measurement purpose of the measure does not need to be 100%. In answering this question, you should evaluate to what extent the measure can be adapted to your needs, or to what extent you and your team can adapt to the measure.

Usefulness of the Measure's Output

How do I intend to use the outcome measure? Can the measure be used this way? These questions about the usefulness of the output of the measure pertain to the relevance of the measure to your quality program. Does the measure give you performance results that you can apply to your efforts to improve nursing care to Alzheimer's patients?

Characteristics of Good Outcome Measures

Now that you have determined that a given measure is of use, you should evaluate key characteristics of the measure to insure that it is defined, tested, and operationalized adequately.

• Targets improvement

The measure and its output must focus on improvement in nursing care not merely on the description of some aspect of care. Having an accurate measure that tells you the status of a given aspect of care is not helpful. Instead, the measure needs to inform you about current quality levels and relate them to previous and future quality levels. The measure needs to compute improvements or declines in quality over time so that you can plan for the future.

• *Precisely defined and specified*

The measure needs to be clearly defined, including the terms used, the data elements collected, and the calculation steps to be made.

• *Validity*

Obtaining information about the validity of a measure is important. Validity refers to whether the measure "actually measures what it purports to measure" [4].

• *Sensitivity and Specificity*

These concepts refer to the measure's ability to capture all true cases of the event being measured, and only true cases. Make sure that an outcome measure identifies true cases as true, and false cases as false, and does not identify a true case as false or a false case as true. Sensitivity of an outcome measure is the likelihood of a positive test when a condition is present. Lack of sensitivity is expressed as "false positives" (ie, the indicator calculates a condition as present when it is not). Specificity refers to the likelihood of a negative test when a condition is not present. "False negatives" reflect lack of specificity (ie, the indicators calculate that a condition is not present when in fact it is).

• *Reliability*

Reliability means that results are reproducible; the indicator measures the same attribute consistently across the same patients and across time. A measure is reliable if different people calculate the same rate for the same patient sample. The core issue of reliability is measurement error, the difference between the actual phenomenon and its measurement (ie, the greater the difference, the less reliable the outcome measure).

• *Interpretable*

An outcome measure must be interpretable; that is, convey a result that can be linked to the quality of nursing care. First, the quantitative output of an outcome measure ("the number you get") must be scaled in such a way that users can interpret it. For instance, a scale that starts with 0 as the lowest possible level and ends with 100 is a lot easier to interpret than a scale that starts with 144 and has no upper boundary except infinity.

• *Risk-adjusted*

Some patients are sicker than others are; some patients have more comorbidities; some patients are older and frailer, and so forth. Certainly, you could come up with many more risk variables that influence how Alzheimer's patients respond to nursing care. Good outcome measures take this differential risk into consideration. They create a "level playing field" by adjusting quality indicators on the basis of the severity of illness, or the risk for the severity of illness, of your patients. Imagine that your patients are a lot sicker than those of another facility to which you are being compared. You and your team are at greater risk for having lower quality outcomes, not because you provide inferior care, but because your patients are a lot sicker to begin with and may not respond as well as less sick patients.

Box 3: Common problems with outcome measures

1. *Lack of focus.* This is a measure that tries to measure too many things at the same time or is too complicated to administer, interpret, or use.

2. *Wrong type of measure.* This is a measure that calculates indicators the wrong way (eg, uses rates when ratios are more appropriate), uses a continuous scale when a discrete scale would be more informative (or vice versa), or measures a process when the outcome is measurable and of greater interest.

3. *Unclear definitions.* This is a measure that is too broad or too vague in its scope and definitions (eg, population is too heterogeneous), no risk adjustment, unclear data elements, or poorly defined values.

4. *Too much work.* This is a measure that requires too much nursing time to generate data or too much manual chart abstraction.

5. *Reinventing the wheel.* It is okay to invent a better wheel by improving the materials, mechanics, and physics of the wheel. Likewise, it is okay to improve an outcome measure; yet, ask yourself, is this really an improvement or just a reinvention?

6. *Measures events not within your control.* You can only change what you do and what you influence. Do not select a measure that focuses on a process or outcome that is out of your control to improve.

7. *Trying to do research rather than quality management.* Research entails data collection and analysis, but not all data collection and analysis is research, nor should it be. Stay focused! Do not try to change the world, which is what researchers claim to do. Instead, change your practice, your nursing care, and the health and well-being of your Alzheimer's patients. You are more likely to succeed in improving the quality of care in your setting than researchers are likely to change the world.

8. *Poor communication of results.* Do you and your colleagues "get it" when you receive the quality of care results? If you do not, it may be that the results are not communicated effectively.

9. *Uninterpretable and underused.* Uninterpretable results elicit responses of "what does this mean?" and "if I don't get it, what can I do with it?". These results are of little relevance to your quality management program. Even worse is the "so what?" response. This means that you do not recognize the value of the measure to improving nursing care.

- *Easy to Collect*

It might be helpful to use outcome measures for which data are readily available, can be retrieved from existing sources, or can be collected with little burden. The goal is to gather good data quickly without running the risk of having "quick-and-dirty" data.

- *Within Your Control*

Outcome measures are indicators of quality. These indicators should reflect nursing practice and can be influenced by nursing care if you propose that they relate to nursing care. You cannot improve quality scores if the measures are based on variables outside your control.

Common Problems with Outcome Measures

Just as much as you evaluate the strengths of an outcome measure, you should review potential weaknesses (Box 3).

Using Existing Measures

Begin the process of deciding how to measure by reviewing existing measures. Reinventing the wheel is unnecessary, especially if good measures are out there. Review the literature, check with national organizations, and consult your colleagues; yet, do not adopt existing measures blindly. Instead, subject them to a thorough review using the characteristics identified above. Also, contact health care organizations that have adopted these measures and review with them their experience.

Developing New Measures

After an exhaustive search, you may not find measures that meet the various requirements outlined above. You decide instead to develop your own in-house measure. The list of good and bad characteristics of outcome measures should guide you and your team in your development efforts (Box 4).

SUMMARY

The process of outcome measurement and quality management in nursing care of Alzheimer's patients is not a mystery. It is hard work identifying what to measure, selecting the measures, collecting the data, analyzing and presenting results, and implementing change. To summarize, when determining the final measures that are good for you and your organization, three things matter:

1. It works for your organization.
2. It is well defined, tested, and applied.
3. Quality improvement happens!

Box 4: Developing new measures

1. *Zero in on the subpopulation to be measured.* If you are measuring an undesirable event, determine the subgroup of Alzheimer's patients at risk for experiencing that event, and limit your denominator population to that group. If you are measuring a desirable event or process, identify the group that should experience the event or receive the process. Where do problems tend to occur? What variables of this problem are within your control?

2. *Define your terms.* This part of the process is a painstaking but essential exercise. Try to be as precise as possible, even if it feels "techy." It is better to measure 80% of an issue with 100% accuracy, than 100% of an issue with 80% accuracy.

3. *Identify the data elements.* Be clear about what you want to measure, how you will measure it, and how you will calculate the performance score, another painstaking but essential effort. The 80/100 rule applies here also.

4. *Test the data collection process.* Once you have a prototype of a measure ready, examine how easy or difficult it is to get all the required data.

References

[1] Institute of Medicine. To err is human: building a safer health system. In: Kohn LT, Corrigan JM, Donaldson MS, editors. Washington, D.C: National Academy Press; 2000.

[2] Schyve PM, Nadzam DM. Outcome measurement in healthcare. Journal of Strategic Outcome Measurement 1998;2(4):34–42.

[3] McGlynn EA, Asch SM. Developing a clinical outcome measure. Am J Prev Med 1998; 14(35):14–21.

[4] Wilson HS. Research in nursing. 2nd edition. Reading (MA): Addison-Wesley; 1989.

Nurs Clin N Am 41 (2006) 105–117

NURSING CLINICS
OF NORTH AMERICA

ELSEVIER
SAUNDERS

Longitudinal Observational Studies to Study the Efficacy-Effectiveness Gap in Drug Therapy: Application to Mild and Moderate Dementia

Karen M. MacDonald, PhD, RN[a],*, Stefaan Vancayzeele, MD[b], Anne Deblander, MD[b], Ivo L. Abraham, PhD, RN, CS, FAAN[a,c,d,e,f]

[a]Matrix45, LLC 620 Frays Ridge Road, Earlysville, VA 22936, USA
[b]Novartis Pharma Belgium, Vilvoorde, Belgium
[c]Center for Health Outcomes and Policy Research, School of Nursing & Leonard Davis Institute of Health Economics, Wharton School of Business, University of Pennsylvania, PA, USA
[d]College of Nursing, University of Arizona, Tucson, AZ, USA
[e]School of Nursing, New York University, New York, NY, USA
[f]School of Nursing, University of Virginia, Charlottesville, VA, USA

Pharmacologic therapies are required to be tested rigorously for safety and efficacy before they can be considered for public use. Although there is a lack of a single, harmonized definition of safety among regulating agencies, safety is related to a drug's risk (or potential) for producing adverse events or reactions (ie, unintended noxious responses) [1]. Efficacy is the extent to which a specific intervention (a drug, in this case) produces a beneficial effect under controlled conditions [2]. The critical studies come in phase 3, after initial safety has been established in phase 1 studies and initial efficacy and additional safety have been examined in phase 2 studies. In phase 3, randomized controlled trials (RCTs) are conducted to establish more definitely the efficacy while continuing to examine the safety of a potential drug [3]. If a drug is found to be efficacious and safe, it is submitted for approval to regulatory agencies. Once approved and marketed, drugs are further assessed (by way of phase 4 studies) for safety and efficacy. Like earlier phases, phase 4 studies are predominately RCTs. Following safety concerns and withdrawal from the market in 2004 of the approved Cox-2 inhibitor analgesic, rofecoxib, drug regulatory agencies are putting in place more stringent requirements for postmarketing drug surveillance and assessment [4].

*Corresponding author. Matrix45, LLC 620 Frays Ridge Road, Earlysville, VA 22936.
E-mail address: kmacdonald@matrix45.com (K.M. MacDonald).

0029-6465/06/$ – see front matter
doi:10.1016/j.cnur.2005.10.002

Although long-term safety is one concern of approved marketed drugs, another important issue is drug effectiveness (ie, whether a drug that has been proven to be safe and efficacious in RCTs actually provides benefit to patients when used in daily practice). Efficacy is the beneficial effect obtained under the controlled conditions of a research setting in selected study subjects, but effectiveness has been defined as the extent to which a specific intervention (ie, a drug) does what it is intended to do when deployed in the field under uncontrolled conditions [2]. Often, and especially in treatment of chronic illnesses, there is an efficacy-effectiveness gap once drugs migrate from RCTs to real-world use. That is, drugs that provide a measurable benefit in controlled (protocol-driven) administration in selected patients often do not produce the same benefit when used to varying degrees in the community in "average" patients.

Practicing clinicians know that in addition to the proven efficacy of a drug, many other contributing factors exist that determine the real-world effectiveness of pharmacologic therapies (eg, the prescribed dose and frequency), whether the patient actually takes the medication, the patient's comorbidities, concomitant medications, and so forth. These real-world variabilities that impact drug effectiveness cannot be randomized and studied by way of traditional clinical trial methods and designs (eg, randomly assigning patients to a noncompliant group, for example, would be unethical). The assessment of the real-world variability that exists at the patient-level, the caregiver/family-level, the provider-level, and even the community-level needs to be conducted through methods that allow for the evaluation of outcomes of these various patient, family, provider, and community factors. The utility of this inquiry lies in identifying (and subsequently targeting) those factors that are modifiable or manageable.

RCTs remain the gold standard for evaluation of drug safety and efficacy. Although they are essential in drug development and drug approval, they are insufficient for determining their real-world effectiveness and must be complemented by other methods of inquiry in the postmarketing, phase 4 evaluation of approved drugs. Longitudinal observational studies (LOSs) offer more than the means to explore and describe; they can provide the methods to evaluate real-world effectiveness of interventions, including pharmacotherapeutics.

Drug therapy for Alzheimer's disease and related dementias is recent, yet patients, families, and advocacy organizations have shown great interest and have lobbied for their approval and reimbursement. Four drugs have been approved in the USA and Europe: tacrine, donepezil, rivastigmine, and galantamine. These drugs have been shown to produce "modest but temporary improvements in cognition, global functioning, activities of daily living, and behavior" and some evidence exists demonstrating that these drugs may delay disease progression slightly [5]. However, ample clinical evidence of variation in outcomes also exists, which makes it more difficult for clinicians, patients, and families to make decisions about treatment. Longitudinal observational studies may assist in better understanding how dementia drugs work over time, the different factors that may influence outcomes, and patients groups that may benefit more than others from these drugs.

If well-designed, LOSs can provide insights to the linkages between real-world outcomes and their multilevel determinants. In this article, some of the scientific and methodologic issues related to LOSs in pharmacotherapeutic evaluations are discussed. A case of such a study in the treatment of mild to moderate dementia is provided—a case in which a pharmaceutic sponsor addressing a medical question (long-term effectiveness) realized that caring for patients who have Alzheimer's disease involves the clinical community of caregivers, physicians, families, nurses, psychologists, and pharmacists, among others, and partnered with nurse researchers to design their inquiry. The authors conclude by presenting an argument for nurses to take the lead in effectiveness research.

LONGITUDINAL OBSERVATIONAL STUDIES IN PHARMACOTHERAPEUTIC EVALUATIONS

Traditionally, most phase 4 drug studies have been RCTs to study formulations, refine dosages and durations of treatment, explore drug-drug interactions, or evaluate use in specific demographic patient groups. Phase 4 studies that are observational or nonexperimental are frequently called postmarketing surveillance and seek to document previously unknown or inadequately quantified adverse reactions and related risk factors. In both cases, the focus has continued to be primarily on safety and efficacy. Observational studies in phase 4 drug evaluations, however, also are being used more frequently to evaluate drug effectiveness—the evaluation of how approved, marketed drugs are used in the real world (ie, how drugs are actually used by typical clinicians in everyday practice in their patient populations).

With rising health care costs increasing pressure exists to reimburse only for services that have not demonstrated only safety and efficacy but also demonstrated effectiveness and cost-effectiveness [6]. Hence, growing incentives exist to conduct effectiveness and pharmaco-economic evaluations of interventions, including pharmaotherapeutics. Longitudinal observational studies, which are much faster and cheaper and more feasible to conduct in large samples, provide a method for achieving these goals.

Considerable debate exists in the clinical research literature in the past decade over the validity of the findings from observational studies. Although evidence exists supporting the validity of well-designed observational studies [7,8], challenges remain in convincing the "RCT-or-bust" critics. This "RCT-or-bust" perspective against LOSs is partly a result of a lack of methodologic sophistication on the part of its critics. This lack is in part because of an unfortunate history of poorly designed LOSs that had little scientific relevance but mainly commercial objectives. The question is not which design is superior but which design is most appropriate for answering a specific set of research questions.

Fig. 1 [9] illustrates the continuum of health-related research. The boundaries between the categories are somewhat artificial and much of contemporary health care research overlaps the categories, whereas the basic distinction is that biomedical research deals with questions of "what causes diseases and

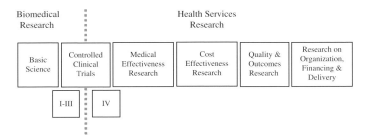

Fig. 1. Continuum of health-related research (*Adapted from* Eisenberg JM. Health services research in a market-oriented health care system. Health Affairs 1998;17:98–108.

how can they be prevented or treated"? Health services research deals with "what works, what does it cost, and how do we close the gap between what we know and what we do?" [9] More specifically, phase 1 through 3 RCTs answer the question, "what interventions can work in certain patients under certain conditions?" Postmarketing studies and other effectiveness and outcomes studies answer the question, "Does it work in the real world – and how?"

In the hierarchy of levels of evidence (Table 1), observational studies fall lower than RCTs or quasi-experimental studies [10,11,12] primarily as a result of the lack of control exerted in the sample selection and in the administration of interventions. Real-world variability (ie, heterogeneity) in patient characteristics and practice patterns (among other things) is precisely what the LOS seeks to identify and evaluate. Lack of control and inclusion of variability in patient and treatment characteristics (and linking those to outcomes) is where the LOS is more powerful in answering questions of effectiveness than the RCT. Although the hierarchy of evidence classifies study designs according to degree of control of extraneous or confounding variables, however, it cannot guide the

Table 1
Example of one classification of hierarchy of evidence

Level	Type of evidence
Ia	Evidence obtained from meta-analysis of randomized controlled trials
Ib	Evidence obtained from at least one randomized controlled trial
II-a	Evidence obtained from at least one well-designed controlled study without randomization
II-b	Evidence obtained from at least one other type of well-designed, quasi-experimental study
III	Evidence obtained from well-designed, nonexperimental descriptive studies, such as comparative studies, correlation studies, and case studies
IV	Evidence obtained from expert committee reports or opinions or clinical experiences of respected authorities

From Clinical practice guideline No.1: acute pain management: operative or medical procedures and trauma; 1993. Rockville (MD): US Department of Health and Human Services. Agency for Health Care Policy and Research, Publication # 92–0023.

determination of appropriateness of study design. Again, the best study design is the one that is most appropriate in answering the question(s) at hand.

The hierarchy of evidence classifications is used to evaluate a body of evidence (ie, all of the existing [or at least published or accessible] research on a particular topic or intervention). This evaluation across all levels of the hierarchy is critical to the development of clinical practice guidelines or best practice guidelines (BPGs). BPGs provide clinicians with concise and easily accessible, evidence-based decision support. BPGs are not intended to replace clinical experience or judgment and do not mandate interventions; rather, they provide recommendations for care under certain scenarios. In essence, the intention of BPGs is to reduce the variability in clinical practice so that patients actually receive "as close to" the standard of care as possible (standard of care being defined as that determined through the available evidence).

Unfortunately, adoption of BPGs by clinicians is mixed and disappointing [13] even though BPGs provide a benchmark against which to evaluate variability in clinical practice patterns and outcomes. The emergence of evidence-based guidelines as the standard of care essentially necessitates the assessment of the extent to which clinicians are practicing in accordance with BPGs and the extent to which BPGs improve patient outcomes. These questions lend themselves to observational study designs (frankly, what patient or clinician, let alone an ethical review board, would find it acceptable in a RCT to be assigned to the other-than-best-practice group?).

Practice patterns are only one source of variability that may alter the real-world effectiveness of drugs that have demonstrated safety and efficacy. No doubt the patient plays a central role, actively and passively, in the determination of outcomes. In addition to patient sociodemographic characteristics, the role of a patient's health beliefs, knowledge (of disease and treatment), health behaviors (health promoting and health damaging), comorbid conditions, concomitant treatments, and treatment adherence (compliance and persistence) all may contribute to treatment effectiveness. Furthermore, family structure and dynamics, in addition to clinician or health care system characteristics, may have an influence. The myriad of factors that determines the effectiveness of drugs used every day in the real world is complex. Subsequently, effectiveness research is challenging and requires the application of methods that go beyond the statistical difference testing that is often used in RCTs. Although RCTs, by design, ensure the benefits and constraints of homogeneity of subjects, LOSs must overcome the challenges of heterogeneity of subjects through identifying confounding variables, application of statistical controls, or post hoc analyses. Some of these methods are illustrated briefly in the case study of the FExT Study being conducted in Belgium.

CASE: THE FEXT STUDY IN BELGIUM—UNDERSTANDING PRACTICE PATTERNS, DETERMINANTS, AND OUTCOMES

Rivastigmine tartrate is a potent, dual cholinesterase (ChE) inhibitor indicated for the symptomatic treatment of patients with mild to moderately severe

Alzheimer's disease. The efficacy of rivastigmine tartrate treatment has been demonstrated in large, randomized, placebo-controlled clinical trials involving more than 3300 patients with mild to moderately severe Alzheimer's disease [14]. Rivastigmine tartrate provides significant clinical efficacy across all three key symptom domains of Alzheimer's disease: activities of daily living, behavioral and psychological symptoms of dementia, and cognition. The improvements in behavior, including psychotic symptoms, have reduced the need for psychotropic agents, including antipsychotics, in open-label studies in nursing home patients [15,16,17]. Of note are data from recent studies, which suggest that rivastigmine tartrate slows disease progression in Alzheimer's patients [18,19]. In placebo-controlled clinical trials with open-label extensions, patients who started on placebo then switched to rivastigmine tartrate never "caught up" with those patients who received continuous rivastigmine tartrate therapy.

With the efficacy of rivastigmine established in key trials, it is now important to examine the actual patterns of use of rivastigmine and other drugs in its class, link these patterns to direct yet broader outcomes in patients, and examine corollary outcomes in primary caregivers. Thus, it is critical to complement prior trials on the efficacy of rivastigmine with observational, epidemiologic studies that evaluate variations in the "real-world" management of patients' cognitive, behavioral, and functional deficits associated with Alzheimer's disease. Further, and in light of the recent recommendations from the Agency for Health care Quality and Research's 2004 *Evidence Report on Pharmacological Treatment of Dementia* [20], additional research is needed related to the effects of treatments on the burden of caregivers of patients with Alzheimer's disease. A better understanding of the multitude of real-world factors at the patient- and caregiver-level, the provider-level, and the practice-level that are associated with the outcomes of treatment with rivastigmine may enable clinicians to modify practices to better achieve treatment goals.

Consequently, Novartis Pharma Belgium is conducting an observational, pharmaco-epidemiologic study to evaluate the multilevel factors and outcomes in the daily practice of managing the cognitive, functional, and behavioral deficits of patients with mild to moderate Alzheimer's disease and their primary caregivers' sense of burden and stress. See Fig. 2 for a framework of the clinical and scientific issues that served as drivers for the planning of this initiative and the major goals of this LOS and the corresponding analytic techniques. The combination of this study's findings with those from clinical trials and other observational studies enables a better understanding of the "real world" determinants of clinical response to rivastigmine and builds an evidence-based approach to treatment, caregiver services, medical education, and clinician support. The authors briefly describe the objectives and key aspects of the methods of this on-going study.

Study Objectives

The general aim of this study is to examine the multilevel (patient and caregiver level, physician level [general practitioner and specialist], and practice level)

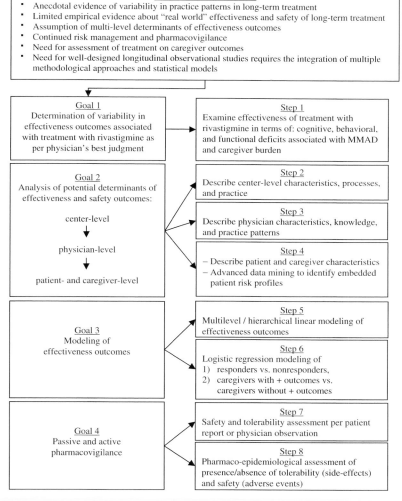

Fig. 2. Study framework: drivers, goals, and analytical procedures.

determinants and outcomes of rivastigmine, a pseudo-irreversible cholinesterase inhibitor, in the cognitive, behavioral, and functional management of patients with mild to moderate Alzheimer's disease (MMAD). As the management of patients with Alzheimer's disease closely involves the primary caregiver and the family at large, this study considers caregiver- and family-related variables as mediators of patient outcomes but also as direct outcomes; and will be studied within the same multilevel framework.

This study has enrolled rivastigmine-naïve patients who are started on rivastigmine per their prescribing physician's decision for the treatment of MMAD. The patient-level outcomes include:

- Cognitive status as measured by the Mini-Mental State Exam (MMSE [21])
- Overall status and deterioration as measured by the Global Deterioration Scale (GDS [22])
- Physical activities of daily living as measured by the Katz ADL scale (ADL [23])
- Instrumental activities of daily living as measured by the Lawton IADL scale (IADL [24])
- Behavioral status as measured by the Neuropsychiatric Inventory (NPI [25]).

These variables are considered positive if levels are the same or improved at 6 or 12 months related to baseline.

The patient's primary caregiver completes a self-reported survey comprised of demographic data and the following outcome variables:

- Instrumental activities of daily living by way of the Lawton IADL scale
- Perceived burden of caregiving as measured by the Caregiver Burden Scale [26]
- Psychologic distress as measured by the 12-item General Health Questionnaire (GHQ-12 [27,28]).

Positive caregiver outcome is defined as the reduction in caregiver burden and stress levels at 6 or 12 months compared with that caregiver's baseline levels; or, if low baseline levels, the maintenance of these low levels at 6 or 12 months. Patients' and caregivers' perceptions of and satisfaction with treatment also are evaluated.

Data are collected on characteristics of the patient's general practitioner and their specialist physician initiating rivastigmine treatment. This information includes general demographic data and data related to their length of practice experience and certification or accreditation. More specific information related to the management of patients who have dementia are collected (volume, frequency, duration of office visits by patients who have dementia, and approach to management of dementia). Physicians are queried about their customary sources of information/knowledge on dementia and Alzheimer's disease and their understanding of standards of care and consensus positions. Generalists and specialists provide data on their preferred prescribing patterns for dementia, including initiation of treatment, intensification of treatment, management of side effects, and patient drug compliance.

Research Questions and Significance

Several research questions guide this LOS and are listed below, along with an explanation of the answers being sought and why these are important.

1. *Can two or more clusters of MMAD patients being evaluated for MMAD and being considered for treatment with rivastigmine be identified, quantified, tested for difference, and described in clinical terms? The knowledge base*

about some diseases and their associated etiology, explicit risks factors, and explicit characteristics is extensive and patients can be easily classified according to defined taxonomies or risk profiles; however, the explanatory value of those risk classifications may be focused too much on explicit or "surface" variability. Therefore, deeply embedded and implicit profiles that may aid in better understanding the interface between patient and treatment should be examined. In many cases, the state of the science lacks such understanding. Advanced data mining statistical methods can be used to identify risk subcohorts or "clusters" of patients. These methods attempt to reveal associations and discover structures in data that may not have been previously evident but that are meaningful and useful once found. Although data mining methods may not always provide an explanation or interpretation as to why risk groupings of patients exist, they can identify clusters of patients who share similar attributes along a set of parameters and thus may be useful in identifying patients at risk for poor outcomes. In this study, parameters are specified a priori based on extant studies, clinical experience, and exploratory analysis of potentially relevant variables in the study database (eg, demographic factors, medical history, living conditions, and caregiver/family support). If profiles are meaningful, useful, and definable in clinical terms, profiles will be tested in subsequent analyses to determine if they can differentiate patients on treatment outcomes.

2. *How are patient-, caregiver-, physician-, and practice-level variables, independently or in interaction, related to patient and caregiver outcomes in patients who have MMAD (entire sample and within each cluster); and how do these variables explain the variance in observed outcomes?* The examination of the multilevel determinants (at the patient-, caregiver-, physician- and practice-level) of patient outcomes and caregiver outcomes is central to the effectiveness evaluation of treatment with rivastigmine. Multilevel, or hierarchical, modeling enables the assessment of not only patient-level characteristics as determinants of patient outcomes but also the assessment of caregiver-, physician-, and practice-level characteristics as determinants of patient outcomes (the same is true for caregiver outcomes). Using these methods, not only is the contribution of specific variables to the outcome determined (similar to other modeling techniques), but the amount of variability in the outcome that is attributable to each level, or class, can be computed through the intraclass correlation coefficient (ICC). As each participating center contributes several physicians and each physician contributes several patients to this study, patients are not independent but considered "nested" under physicians who are likewise "nested" under centers. Thus, all patients recruited by one physician are assumed to share some proportion of variance in outcome that might be attributable to their common treating physician *prior* to any patient-specific determinants of variability (and the same for variance attributable to center effects). The ICC (which can range from .00 to 1.00; convertible to 0% to 100%) quantifies the variability in patient outcome that is attributable to within-physician variability. Thus, the ICC quantifies the overall magnitude of the class effect. The ICC is computed for each level and the sum of ICCs for all levels equals 1.00. Such an understanding of the magnitude of the class effect and the contribution of specific, multilevel determinants to patient outcomes and caregiver outcomes (in the sample as

a whole and in the clusters identified under Question 1) will assist clinicians in targeting factors that are modifiable or manageable.

3. *Are there differences in patient-, caregiver-, physician-, and practice-level variables, independently or in interaction, between 1) responders and nonresponders to treatment with rivastigmine in the management of MMAD,[a] and 2) caregivers with positive outcomes and those without positive outcomes?* Similar to research Question 2, the modeling of the contributing factors to successful treatment versus unsuccessful treatment is an essential part of the effectiveness evaluation. In this case, logistic regression is used to model the multilevel determinants of patient outcomes and caregiver outcomes after classifying patients and caregivers to dichotomous outcome groups: responder/nonresponder and positive/negative, respectively.

The inclusion of such various and numerous determinant and outcome variables, as is typical in LOSs, and the methods used to evaluate them require large sample sizes of patients. If, as in this Belgian study, a LOS intends to study determinants beyond the patient (eg, caregiver-level, physician-level, and so forth), it is essential to recruit sufficient numbers of clinicians and centers. Therefore, the FExT study is a multicenter study with a target sample size to 642 patients recruited from at least 70 practices. Once recruited into the study, patients are asked to revisit the specialist physician approximately 6 and 12 months after their first visit.

At the time of this publication, data collection for the FExT study is nearing completion. It is anticipated that, regardless of any specific findings (in terms of direction, magnitude, or significance) related to patient profiling, the associations between determinants and outcomes, and differences in the determinants between those successfully treated and those not successfully treated, the wealth of previously unavailable information obtained from this LOS will shed new light on the daily, real-world use of rivastigmine in patients with Alzheimer's disease. While there are, no doubt, determinants that are beyond the manipulation or control of the patients, caregivers, or physicians, this new information has the potential to provide insights and understanding of some determinants that may be modifiable or manageable.

Informed Consent

The issue of informed consent is particularly important when studying vulnerable patients, such as those with dementia—even in noninterventional studies. Patients should be fully informed of the study purpose; methods of the study, including duration, treatments, and assessments; nature of the commitment from subject's point of view (eg, number and timing of follow-up visits and assessments); potential risks and benefits of participation; costs (including time

---

[a]A treatment responder is a patient who meets the following three conditions: (1) persistence on rivastigmine for at least 6 months, with titration per physician's decision after at any time during up to 12 months; (2) no subjective drug intolerance, as measured by patient willingness to continue rivastigmine treatment for at least 6 months; (3). MMSE levels either same at 6 or 12 months relative to baseline; or improved at 6 or 12 months relative to baseline; or declined but with lesser negative slope at 6 or 12 months than known decline slope of untreated patients.

and travel) and compensation (if any) of participation; data handling including confidentiality/anonymity; contact information of the investigator and investigating institution; and the voluntary nature of their participation, that is, their right to refuse to participate or to withdraw later without consequences. If patients are incapable of comprehending the issues or are not competent to give informed consent, then the patient's legal guardian can, if fully informed, provide consent. Whether obtained from the patient or the legal guardian, consent to participate should be obtained free from coercion and undue influence. They should be provided assurances that their decision (either way) will not affect their access to care or their relationship with their care providers. In the FExT study, where many patients experience only mild dementia, the determination of competence to consent is made by the physician. In addition to patient or legal guardian consent for patient participation, the consent of the caregiver is necessary for their participation.

NURSING AND EFFECTIVENESS RESEARCH: WHY NURSES SHOULD TAKE THE LEAD

The effectiveness evaluation of pharmaceutical products no doubt requires the collaboration of a multidisciplinary team. An argument exists, however, for not merely the participation of nurses on such teams but for nurse researchers to actually lead effectiveness research. The distinction should be made between the role of research nurses and the role of nursing research. The former involves clinical or research staff to screen and enroll patients, provide patient education and obtain informed consent, conduct assessments and administer interventions as appropriate, and ensure adherence to proper data collection procedures. The latter involves the participation in the conceptualization of the study (development and articulation of strategic, clinical, and scientific drivers and questions), selection of appropriate study design and methods to answer the identified study questions (including assurance of inclusion of relevant factors in the data model), participation in development of the analytic plan, and the critical role in the interpretation and translation of the findings for dissemination.

The argument for nurses to lead effectiveness research lies in the pivotal and central role of nurses in the day-to-day conduct of health care delivery in the real world. Nursing issues deal with and nurses spend most of their time in direct contact with patients and caregivers in the provision of patient and family support (ie, holistic care of the patient not just treatment of the disease); education of disease and treatments; assessments, education, and interventions for prevention and health promotion; and education and strategies for enhancing patient compliance. Furthermore, nurses interface with and often coordinate the care provided from all other facets of the health care system—physicians, pharmacists, psychologists, social workers, and so forth (in addition to frequently having knowledge of or responsibilities for administrative and reimbursement issues and procedures). Thus, nurses have intimate knowledge of patient-related factors and other multilevel factors that potentially may contribute, positively and adversely, to drug effectiveness. In a way, effectiveness research deals with issues that have always been central to nursing.

Effectiveness research is complementary to efficacy and safety research as much as nursing research is complementary to biomedical research. Efficacy and safety studies, although necessary for drug development and approval, are not sufficient for determining real-world effectiveness. In this regard, effectiveness research contributes to advancing understanding and to improving patient care.

References

[1] ICH harmonised tripartite guideline. E2A: Clinical safety data management: definitions and standards for expedited reporting. International Conference on Harmonisation of Technical Requirements for Registration of Pharmaceutical for Human Use. Brussels, Belgium; October 27, 1994.

[2] Last JM. A dictionary of epidemiology. 2nd edition. Oxford (UK): Oxford University Press; 1988.

[3] Guidance for industry: premarketing risk assessment. US Department of Health and Human Services. Food and Drug Administration. Center for Drug Evaluation and Research. Rockville, (MD); 2005.

[4] Guidance for industry: good pharmacovigilance practices and pharmacoepidemiologic assessment. Rockville (MD): US Department of Health and Human Services. Food and Drug Administration. Center for Drug Evaluation and Research. 2005.

[5] Hake AM, Farlow MR. On the horizon: pathways for drug development in Alzheimer's disease. Clin Geriatr Med 2004;20(1):141–52.

[6] Ruchlin HS, Dasbach EJ, Heyse JF. New directions in pharmacoeconomic research: the next step. Drug Inf J 2002;36:909–17.

[7] Benson K, Hartz A. A comparison of observational studies and randomized, controlled trials. N Engl J Med 2000;342:1878–86.

[8] Concato J, Shah N, Horwitz R. Randomized, controlled trials, observational studies and the hierarchy of research designs. N Engl J Med 2000;342:1887–92.

[9] Eisenberg JM. Health services research in a market-oriented health care system. Health Aff 1998;17:98–108.

[10] Clinical practice guideline No. 1: acute pain management: operative or medical procedures and trauma; 1993. Rockville (MD): US Department of Health and Human Services. Agency for Health Care Policy and Research, Publication # 92–0023.

[11] Hadorn DC, Baker D, Hodges JS, et al. Rating the quality if evidence for clinical practice guidelines. J Clin Epidemiol 1996;49(7):749–54.

[12] United States preventive services task force. Guide to clinical preventive services. 2nd edition. Baltimore (MD): Williams & Wilkins; 1996.

[13] Timmermans S, Mauck A. The Promises and pitfalls of evidence-based medicine. Health Aff 2005;24:18–28.

[14] Schneider LS, Anand R, Farlow MR. Systematic review of the efficacy of rivastigmine for patients with Alzheimer's disease. Int J Geriatr Psychopharmacol 1998;1:S26–34.

[15] Cummings J, Anand R, Koumaras B, et al. Rivastigmine provides behavioral benefits to Alzheimer's disease patients residing in a nursing home: findings from a 56-week trial. Neurology 2000;54(Suppl 3):A468–9.

[16] Bullock R, Moulias R, Steinwachs KC, et al. Effects of rivastigmine on behavioural symptoms in nursing home patients with Alzheimer's disease. Int Psychogeriatr 2001;13(Suppl 2): 242. Abstract P-248.

[17] Etemad B. Behavioral and cognitive benefits of rivastigmine in nursing home patients with Alzheimer's disease and related dementias: a 26-week follow-up. Int Psychogeriatr 2001;13(Suppl 2):241. Abstract P-246.

[18] Farlow MR, Hake A, Messina J, et al. The response of patients with Alzheimer's disease to rivastigmine treatment is predicted by the rate of disease progression. Arch Neurol 2001;58:417–22.

[19] Rösler M, Retz W, Retz-Junginger P, et al. Effects of two-year treatment with the cholinester-ase inhibitor rivastigmine on behavioural symptoms in Alzheimer's disease. Behav Neurol 1998;11:211–6.

[20] Santaguida PS, Raina P, Booker L, et al. Pharmacological treatment of dementia. Evidence report/technology assessment No. 97; 2004 (prepared by McMaster University Evidence-Based Practice Center under Contract No. 290–02–0020). Rockville (MD): Agency for Healthcare Research and Quality, Publication #04–E018–2.

[21] Folstein M, Folstein SE, McHugh PR. "Mini-Mental State": a practical method for grading the cognitive state of patients for the clinician. J Psychiatr Res 1975;12(3):189–98.

[22] Reisberg B, Ferris SH, de Leon MJ. The Global Deterioration Scale for assessment of primary degenerative dementia. Am J Psychiatry 1982;139(9):1136–9.

[23] Katz S, Ford AB, Moskowitz RW, et al. Studies of illness in the aged: the index of ADL: a stan-dardized measure of biological and psychosocial function. JAMA 1963;185:914–9.

[24] Lawton MP, Brody EM. Assessment of older people: self-maintaining and instrumental activ-ities of daily living. Gerontologist 1969;9(3):179–86.

[25] Cummings JL, Mega M, Gray K, et al. The Neuropsychiatric Inventory: comprehensive assessment of psychopathology in dementia. Neurology 1994;44(12):2308–14.

[26] Zarit SH, Reever KE, Bach-Peterson J. Relatives of the impaired elderly: correlates of feelings of burden. Gerontologist 1980;20:649–55.

[27] Goldberg D. General Health Questionnaire (GHQ-12). Windsor (UK): NFER-Nelson; 1992.

[28] Pevalin DJ. Multiple applications of the GHQ-12 in a general population sample: an inves-tigation of long-term retest effects. Soc Psychiatry Psychiatr Epidemio 2000;35:508–12.

Nurs Clin N Am 41 (2006) 119–127

NURSING CLINICS
OF NORTH AMERICA

Dementia and Alzheimer's Disease: A Practical Orientation

Ivo L. Abraham, PhD, RN, CS, FAAN[a,b,c,d,e,*]

[a]Matrix45, 620 Frays Ridge Road, Earlysville, VA 22936, USA
[b]Center for Health Outcomes and Policy Research,
School of Nursing and Leonard Davis Institute of Health Economics,
Wharton School of Business, University of Pennsylvania, Philadelphia, PA, USA
[c]College of Nursing, University of Arizona, Tucson, AZ, USA
[d]School of Nursing, New York University, New York, NY, USA
[e]School of Nursing, University of Virginia, Charlottesville, VA, USA

Learning about the essentials of Alzheimer's disease (AD) and related dementias and to differentiate them from other syndromes with seemingly similar symptoms can be a daunting task. In the past 25 years, an explosion has occurred in research and clinical attention to AD, bringing the disease from the sphere of hidden embarrassment to the forefront of clinical care of older adults. Whether one searches the literature or the Internet, one faces massive if not overwhelming amounts of information. Further, much of this information will be put together in function of the target audience and the underlying purpose: patient and family support, clinician education across various disciplines, basic and applied research, to name the major categories. In the end, filtering and synthesizing are essential.

This article aims to provide nurses with a filtered synthesis of *basic* information about AD and related dementias. The focus is on the *essential* and the *practical*: core principles in function of clinical nursing practice. The goal is *not* to provide a comprehensive review of the clinical science and practice of AD but a practical orientation to the basics from a nursing framework, many of which may have become buried in the knowledge explosion of the past 25 years. For a comprehensive review of scientific and clinical issues in AD and dementia, the author refers to Geldmacher [1]. For a more applied text, including practical information for patient and caregiver education and intervention, and family support, a recent publication sponsored by the American Academy of Neurology is recommended highly [2]. These texts complement each other well, though nursing-specific content may not always be evident. Additionally, because AD is no longer a "community" or "nursing home" issue but

*Matrix45, 620 Frays Ridge Road, Earlysville, VA 22936. *E-mail address*: iabraham@matrix45.com

0029-6465/06/$ – see front matter
doi:10.1016/j.cnur.2005.10.001

permeates the entire spectrum of care environments of nurses, it is essential to bring together essential knowledge so nurses can build a foundation for further learning.

DEMENTIA: A CLASS OF BRAIN DISEASE

AD is a form of dementia, and it might be helpful first to review dementia and then to place AD within this disease class. Dementia is "a structurally caused permanent or progressive decline in several dimensions of intellectual function that interferes substantially with the person's normal social and economic activity" [3]. In essence, dementia is the abnormal and gradual decline of several mental functions in later life, and the concurrent decline in one's ability to function independently on a daily basis. Dementia is abnormal and must be differentiated from normal age-related changes in cognition (eg, benign forgetfulness), emotion (eg, heightened vigilance, coping with late life), behavior (eg, structured implementation of activities), and function (eg, some impairment in performing certain activities of daily living because of age-related loss of motor function). Dementia has a gradual onset from initially mild symptoms to more severe symptoms to total impairment in cognition, behavior, emotion, and function. Though dementia in itself does not cause death, the severe decline in all human dimensions is believed to accelerate death (Box 1).

Box 1: What key functions does dementia disrupt?

- *Memory.* Increased forgetfulness evolves into marked impairment in short- and medium-term memory, though some degree of long-term memory may remain. In the initial stages, it is not uncommon for patients to try masking their memory loss by confabulating.

- *Orientation.* This disruption typically starts with disorientation as to time and evolves gradually to disorientation as to place and person.

- *Information processing.* The ability to deal with multiple stimuli in one's environment declines as the disease progresses. Initially, reduced stimulus sets can still be processed, yet at later stages even simple stimulus sets pose a major problem.

- *Problem-solving.* Along with the declining ability to process information, patients become increasingly incapable of making rational decisions. Patients may make strange (irrational) decisions and eventually become unable to make decisions.

- *Judgment.* Judgments about appropriateness and inappropriateness, right and wrong, become increasingly impaired.

- *Sequencing of tasks.* Patients gradually loose the ability to organize actions into a task (eg, the various actions involved in getting dressed).

- *Recognition and naming of objects.* From misrecognition and misnaming to lack of recognition and naming ability.

- *Writing and drawing.* Beginning with impaired writing and drawing ability, this may evolve complete loss of these functions.
- *Calculating.* Incorrect calculation progresses toward inability to perform even simple calculations.
- *Activities of daily living.* Instrumental activities of daily living decline first, but gradually physical activities of daily living are impaired. This disruption may lead to complete dependence upon others for essential tasks, such as eating, dressing, hygiene, going to the bathroom, and other activities.
- *Mood and affect.* Patients may exhibit suppression and excitation of mood and affect—disinterest, restlessness, anxiety, and so forth.
- *Perception and thinking.* Patients who present with dementia may experience hallucinations (perceptions of stimuli that are not present) (eg, hearing voices, seeing things) and delusions (thoughts and beliefs that are not congruent with reality but are real to the patient) (eg, paranoia).
- *Decorum.* Patients gradually lose interest in and control over their appearance, social manners, and language.
- *Behavioral and sexual disinhibition.* Along with the loss of judgment, patients exhibit inappropriate verbal and physical behaviors, with increasing likelihood of various forms of aggression in later stages of the disease. Included here may also be behaviors, such as catastrophic reactions (responses that are disproportionate in intensity to the stimuli that elicited them), wandering (moving around seemingly without purpose), and sundowning (agitation later in the day). Sexual disinhibition, in words and in acts, is not uncommon.
- *Sleep-wake cycle.*

Dementia is an umbrella term for various diseases of the human brain, which express themselves in some configuration of the signs and symptoms described above. The course of dementia differs from patient to patient in signs and symptoms, intensity, and evolution over time.

The various dementias (see later discussion) are often detected too late. Early detection is of critical importance. Table 1 presents a helpful checklist to use in clinical practice when meeting with caregivers and family members [4].

What causes dementia and can different types of dementia be differentiated based on these causes?

> *Plaques and tangles.* A first cause is the degeneration and subsequent death of nerve cells or neurons as happens in AD (which accounts for about 60% of all dementias). This loss of neurons comes from two types of lesions: plaques and tangles. Because of abnormal protein metabolism, deposits of amyloid (plaques) and tangled bundles of fibers (neurofibrillary tangles) develop in the brain, leading to the death of brain cells. Alzheimer's dementia, then, is "a progressive neuropsychiatric disease of aging found in middle-aged and, particularly, in older adults affecting brain matter and characterized by the inexorable loss of cognitive function as well as affective and behavioral disturbances" [5].

Table 1
Checklist for early detection of dementia
Instructions: Based on your family member's behavior in the last two months, please check "yes" or "no" in response to each question below. If you do not understand a question, please check "unsure." Use the "highest concern" column to check the three behaviors that concern you the most.

Have you observed any of the following?	Yes	No	Unsure	Highest concern
Does the person often repeat himself or herself or ask the same questions over and over?				
Is the person more forgetful, such as missing appointments or forgetting conversations?				
Does the person lose things often, such as keys, purse, important papers, or money etc.?				
Does the person need reminders to do things like chores, shopping, or taking medicine?				
Does the person lose track of thoughts in a conversation or have trouble remembering words?				
Does he or she seem sad, down in the dumps, or cry more often than in the past?				
Has he or she started having trouble doing math, paying bills, or keeping a checkbook?				
Does he or she seem less interested in family activities, social activities, or hobbies?				
Have you noticed changes in personal hygiene, dressing, bathing, or using the bathroom?				
Has he or she become irritable, angry, agitated, or suspicious?				
Has he or she started seeing, hearing, or believing things that are not real?				
Has he or she had a personality change, such as saying hurtful things or acting inappropriately?				
Are you concerned about his or her driving, or has he or she stopped driving?				
Are you concerned about his or her judgment, such as trusting strangers, recklessly spending money, or making decisions that are not consistent with his or her previous behavior?				
Does he or she have difficulty operating simple household appliances (eg, the oven, thermostat, remote control, microwave, or telephone?)				
Does he or she become upset, anxious, or nervous, especially when separated from family?				
Does he or she sometimes seem confused by time (eg, confusing night and day or frequently misjudging how much time has elapsed?)				

Adapted from Mundt JC, Freed DM, Griest JH. Lay person-based screening for elderly detection of Alzheimer's disease; development and validation of an instrument. J Gerontol B Psychol Soc Sci 2000;55B:153–70. Adapted, compiled, and expanded by Kate Barrett, LCSW, Orange County Department on Aging with consultation from D. Kaufer, MD, UNC Memory Disorders Clinic, Chapel Hill, NC, 2004.

Lewy bodies and neurites. Also a result of abnormal protein metabolism, Lewy bodies are rounded elements composed of the protein alpha-synuclein found in the cytoplasm of neurons. Lewy neurites contain the same protein but are long in shape. Dementia with Lewy bodies is a neurodegenerative dementia with clinical and pathologic characteristics also seen in Parkinson's disease and AD: cognitive failure; impairments in attention, visual recognition and construction, often fluctuating; and hallucinations [6].

Impaired blood supply to the brain. Occlusion of blood vessels in the brain impairs the flow of blood to and throughout the various parts of the brain and results in localized infarcts and brain cell death. Patients suffer multiple "mini-strokes" (ischemic type) over time, leading to more and more lesions in the brain. This type of dementia is referred to as vascular or multi-infarct dementia [7].

Other brain diseases. Dementia may occur in conjunction with Parkinson's disease, Creutzfeldt-Jacob disease, Pick's disease, nonspecific degeneration in frontal and temporal brain lobes, brain tumors, normal pressure hydrocephalus, and brain trauma secondary to accident [1,6].

Other diseases. Dementia also has been observed in patients who have thyroid disease, vitamin B12 deficiency, alcohol abuse, untreated diabetes, infection, syphilis, and human immodeficiency virus (HIV)/acquired immunodeficiency virus [1,6].

With so many diseases and causes that all express themselves in variations of signs and symptoms, it is not surprising that clinical diagnosis is difficult. As AD received such (much needed) intensive attention from the 1980s on, some "overdiagnosis" of AD and "misdiagnosis" of other types of dementia may have occurred. Regardless, AD remains the most common type of dementia and warrants specific attention.

ALZHEIMER'S DISEASE

AD is not a new disease, only a disease that has become more prevalent with the aging of the population. As a disease of late life, it took increases in longevity as achieved in the second half of the twentieth century to gain more experience with diagnosis and management.

The disease was first described in 1907 by the German neuropathologist Alois Alzheimer who observed the presence of plaques and tangles in the brain of deceased adults who had exhibited a similar pattern of cognitive, emotional, and behavioral impairment. Because the autopsies involved adults younger than 65 years of ago, AD was long believed to be a disease of adulthood not of late life. Only as autopsy results of elderly patients became available and plaques and tangles were observed in them also, did it become evident that AD is a disease of aging and late life.

The epidemiology of AD remains somewhat contested [8], mainly because of differences in study methodologies; however, as a rule of thumb, one can assume that 10% of the population that is 65 years of age and older may suffer from AD—about 5% of those between 65 and 74 years old, almost 20% of those between 75 and 84 years old, and up to 50% of those 85 years and older [9].

Box 2: Checklist developed by the Alzheimer's Association for early detection

1. **Memory loss.** One of the most common early signs of dementia is forgetting recently learned information. Although it is normal to forget appointments, names, or telephone numbers, those with dementia forget these things more often and do not remember them later.

2. **Difficulty performing familiar tasks.** People who have dementia often find it hard to complete everyday tasks that are so familiar others usually do not think about how to do them. A person who has AD may not know the steps for preparing a meal, using a household appliance, or participating in a lifelong hobby.

3. **Problems with language.** Everyone has trouble finding the right word sometimes, but a person who has AD often forgets simple words or substitutes unusual words, making his or her speech or writing hard to understand. If a person who has AD is unable to find his or her toothbrush, for example, the individual may ask for "that thing for my mouth."

4. **Disorientation to time and place.** It is normal to forget the day of the week or where you are going. But people who have AD can become lost on their own street. They may forget where they are and how they got there and may not know how to get back home.

5. **Poor or decreased judgment.** No one has perfect judgment all of the time. Those who have AD may dress without regard to the weather, wearing several shirts on a warm day or little clothing in cold weather. Those who have dementia often show poor judgment about money, giving away large sums to telemarketers, or paying for home repairs or products they do not need.

6. **Problems with abstract thinking.** Balancing a checkbook is a task that can be challenging for some. But a person who has AD may forget what the numbers represent and what needs to be done with them.

7. **Misplacing things.** Anyone can misplace a wallet or key temporarily. A person who has AD may put things in unusual places, like an iron in the freezer or a wristwatch in the sugar bowl.

8. **Changes in mood or behavior.** Everyone can become sad or moody from time to time. Someone who has AD can show rapid mood swings — from calm to tears to anger — for no apparent reason.

9. **Changes in personality.** Personalities ordinarily change somewhat with age. But a person who has AD can change dramatically, becoming extremely confused, suspicious, fearful, or dependent on a family member.

10. **Loss of initiative.** It is normal to tire of housework, business activities, or social obligations at times. The person who has AD may become passive, sitting in front of the television for hours, sleeping more than usual, or not wanting to do usual activities.

If you recognize any warning signs in yourself or a loved one, the Alzheimer's Association recommends consulting a physician.

Reprinted with permission of the Alzheimer's Association.

Box 3: Criteria for Alzheimer's type dementia and age-related cognitive decline

I. Diagnostic criteria for dementia of the Alzheimer's type

A. The development of multiple cognitive deficits manifested by both

1. Memory impairment (impaired ability to learn new information or to recall previously learned information)

2. One (or more) of the following cognitive disturbances:

a. Aphasia (language disturbance)

b. Apraxia (impaired ability to carry out motor activities despite intact motor function)

c. Agnosia (failure to recognize or identify objects despite intact sensory function)

d. Disturbance in executive functioning (ie, planning, organizing, sequencing, abstracting)

B. The cognitive deficits in Criteria A1 and A2 each cause significant impairment in social or occupational functioning and represent a significant decline from a previous level of functioning.

C. The course is characterized by gradual onset and continuing cognitive decline.

D. The cognitive deficits in Criteria A1 and A2 are not caused by any of the following:

1. Other central nervous system conditions that cause progressive deficits in memory and cognition (eg, cerebrovascular disease, Parkinson's disease, Huntington's disease, subdural hematoma, normal-pressure hydrocephalus, brain tumor)

2. Systemic conditions known to cause dementia (eg, hypothyroidism, vitamin B12 or folic acid deficiency, niacin deficiency, hypercalcemia, neurosyphilis, HIV infection)

3. Substance-induced conditions

E. The deficits do not occur exclusively during the course of a delirium.

F. The disturbance is not better accounted for by another Axis I disorder (eg, major depressive disorder, schizophrenia).

II. Description of the condition "age-related cognitive decline"

This category can be used when the focus of clinical attention is an objectively identified decline in cognitive functioning consequent to the aging process that is within normal limits given the person's age. Individuals with this condition may report problems remembering names or appointments or may experience difficulty in solving complex problems. This category should be considered only after it has been determined that the cognitive impairment is not attributable to a specific mental disorder or neurologic condition.

Another helpful rule of thumb is that one third of women and one fifth of men age 65 years or older develop dementia during their lifetime [10]. By 2050, the number of patients who have AD is expected to quadruple [11].

As with dementia, early detection and diagnosis is critical. The Alzheimer's Association has published a checklist of common signs and symptoms to help people recognize the warning signs of AD (Box 2) [12].

The DSM-IV [13] provides several definitions of AD, based on whether the onset is early or late and presence or absence of delirium, delusions, or depressed mood. Box 3 summarizes the DSM-IV criteria.

Box 4: Model for progression of Alzheimer 's disease emphasizing changes and losses

Stage 1 is characterized by

- Initial memory loss impacting patients' hitherto routine activities (work, household, hobbies, social activities, and so forth)
- Forgetting the (ie, being unable to) name of common objects
- Difficulty recognizing and applying numbers (including performing calculations)
- Difficulty processing complex stimulus sets
- Difficulty planning and executing activities
- Difficulty making decisions and solving problems
- Declining interest in habitual and routine activities
- Loss of decorum, initially in dressing and presentation
- Inability to perform instrumental activities of daily living
- Emerging inability to perform selected physical activities of daily living

In Stage 2 patients show, in addition to the above

- Continued memory loss
- Impaired ability to recognize and name familiar people (family and friends)
- Aimless wandering
- Increasing loss of orientation to time, place, and self
- Getting lost in previously familiar environments
- Hallucinations and delusions
- Insomnia and other sleep-wake cycle disruptions

Stage 3 is typified by all of the above and

- Complete memory loss
- Inability to recognize closest family members
- Loss of comprehension of words
- Difficulty swallowing and eating
- Complete dependence on others for physical activities of daily living

The cause or causes of AD remain largely unknown. Many associations between potential causes or factors and the occurrence of AD have been identified. AD, like dementia, is likely an umbrella term for different variants of "plaques and tangles disease": genetic mutation, genetic predisposition, neurotransmitter deficits, toxicity and environmental exposure, autoimmune processes, diet, lifestyle, and so forth. From a nursing perspective, though, this is less relevant as the intensive needs of these patients and their families prevail.

Nurses should understand the progression of the disease. Though various staging models have been proposed, the nursing implications are captured best in a model that emphasizes changes and losses (Box 4).

SUMMARY

This article presents a functional, brief, and, above all, practical orientation to AD. This disease, with its many unanswered questions (and occasional unquestioned answers), is in first instance a disease to be cared for. The burden of this caring initially falls on caregivers and families; however, once Alzheimer's patients enter the formal health care system, nurses will be at the forefront of care. The foundation to good care is a solid but also applied understanding of the disease, how it manifests itself, and how it is experienced by patients, caregivers, and families.

References

[1] Geldmacher DS. Alzheimer's disease and dementia. Clin Geriatr Med 2004;20(1):XI–XII.
[2] Dash P, Villemarette-Pittman N. Alzheimer's disease. New York: Demos Medical Publishers; 2005.
[3] The Merck manual of diagnosis and therapy. 16th edition. Rahway (NJ): Merck & Co; 1992.
[4] Mundt JC, Freed DM, Griest JH. Lay person-based screening for elderly detection of Alzheimer's disease; development and validation of an instrument. J Gerontol B Psychol Soc Sci 2000;55B:153–70.
[5] Butler N. Senile dementia of the Alzheimer's type (SDAT). In: Abrams WB, Berkow R, editors. The Merck manual of geriatarics. Rahway (NJ): Merck & Co; 1990.
[6] McKeith IG, Burn DJ, Ballard CG, et al. Dementia with Lewy bodies. Semin Clin Neuropsychiatry 2003;8(1):46–57.
[7] Sunderland T. Organic brain disorders. In: Abrams WB, Berkow R, editors. The Merck manual of geriatrics. Rahway (NJ): Merck & Co; 1990.
[8] Rocca WA, Hofman A, Brayne C, et al. Frequency and distribution of Alzheimer's disease in Europe: a collaborative study of 1980–1990 prevalence findings. Ann Neurol 1991;30: 381–91.
[9] Evans DA, Funkenstein, Albert MS, et al. Prevalence of Alzheimer's disease in a community population of older persons: higher than previously reported. J Am Med Assoc 1989;262: 2551–9.
[10] Ott A, Breteler MM, van Harskamp F, et al. Incidence and risk of dementia: the Rotterdam study. Am J Epidemiol 1998;147:574–80.
[11] Brookmeyer R, Gray S, Kawas C. Projections of Alzheimer's disease in the United States and the public health impact of delaying disease onset. Am J Public Health 1998;88:1337–42.
[12] Alzheimer's Association. Warning signs of Alzheimer's disease. Available at: http://www.alz.org/AboutAD/Warning.asp. Accessed November 17, 2005.
[13] American Psychiatric Association. Diagnostic and statistical manual of mental disorders. 4th edition. Washington, DC: American Psychiatric Association; 1994.

Nurs Clin N Am 41 (2006) 129

NURSING CLINICS
OF NORTH AMERICA

ELSEVIER
SAUNDERS

Feeding and Hydration Issues for Older Adults with Dementia

Elaine J. Amella, PhD, APRN, BC, FAANP

College of Nursing, Medical University of South Carolina, 99 Jonathan Lucas Street, Charleston, SC 29425, USA

In the *Nursing Clinics of North America*, volume 39, number 3 (September 2004), the article "Feeding and Hydration Issues for Older Adults with Dementia" quoted the Hospice and Palliative Nurses Association (HPNA) position statement on Artificial Nutrition and Hydration (ANH). However, because a sentence was quoted out of context and did not include the entire section, the position of the HPNA is misrepresented. To quote the entire segment:

> The decision to implement ANH should consider probable benefits and burdens of the therapy. Artificial nutrition and hydration has traditionally been used to meet several therapeutic goals: 1) prolong life; 2) prevent aspiration pneumonia; 3) maintain independence and physical function; and 4) decrease suffering and discomfort at the end of life. There are few well-designed studies, however, that have examined whether or not ANH is effective in meeting these goals. The empirical evidence that has been published indicates that ANH often does not affect these clinical objectives (HPNA, 2003).

The editors and author sincerely regret the misrepresentation of the HPNA's position.

Further information is available at http://www.hpna.org/pdf/position_ArtificialNutrition.pdf.

This article refers to doi:10.1016/j.cnur.2004.02.014.

0029-6465/06/$ – see front matter
doi:10.1016/j.cnur.2005.11.002

Nurs Clin N Am 41 (2006) 131–134

INDEX

A

Abuse, of older persons. *See* Elder mistreatment.

Agitation, is assessment of nursing home residents with dementia, 33–34

Alzheimer's Association, checklist for early detection, 126

Alzheimer's disease, abuse and neglect of older adults with, **43–55**
    assessment of, 47–50
    barriers to detection and intervention, 51
    elder mistreatment, 43–44
    prevention and treatment of, 50–51
    reciprocal violence, 46–47
    risk factors for, 44–46
    vulnerability in, 44
  measuring quality of nursing care to patients with, **95–104**
  mild to moderate dementia in, studies of efficacy-effectiveness gap in drug therapy for, **105–117**
  practical orientation to, **119–127**
    checklists for early detection of, 124, 125
    criteria for diagnosis of, 126
    dementia as a class of brain disease, 120–121
    key functions disrupted by dementia in, 122
    model for progression of, 126
  primary care and, issues and challenges in, **83–93**
    clinical dilemmas, 83
    family caregivers, 87, 91
    pharmacologic interventions, 91
    screening, 84–87
    stage-based nursing interventions for, 92–93
    staging, 87, 88–90

Anxiety, in older adults with dementia, 26

Appetite impairment, in older adults with dementia, 26

Assessment, cognitive, in older persons, **1–22**
    conducting the, 3–4
    defining the purpose of, 2
    in delirium, 12–16
    in dementia, 4–8
    in depression, 8–12
    interpreting the results of, 4
    selecting the instrument for, 2–3
  of depression in older adults with dementia, **23–41**
    in nursing home residents, 31–32
    instrumentation as adjunct in, 27–31
  of elder mistreatment and neglect in Alzheimer's patients, 47–50

Assisted living, progressively lowered stress threshold care plan for dementia care in, 64–66

B

Behavioral symptoms, application of progressively lowered stress threshold model in dementia care, **57–81**
  status of, in older patients with dementia, **23–41**
    assessment of depression in nursing homes, 31–32
    behavioral assessment, 32–36
    depression in older adults, key components of, 23–27
      anxiety, 26
      appetite impairment, 26
      disagreeable behavior, 25–26
      lack of meaning in life, 26–27
      melancholic behavior, 25
      sleep impairment, 26
    individualized care for older adults with dementia who are depressed, 32
    instrumentation in assessment of, 27–31
    issues related to, 36–38

C

Caregivers, family, of Alzheimer's patients, 87, 91
    abuse and neglect by, **43–55**
    stage-based nursing interventions for, 92–93

Note: Page numbers of article titles are in **boldface** type.

0029-6465/06/$ – see front matter
doi:10.1016/S0029-6465(06)00022-3

Cognitive assessment, in older persons,
   1–22
        conducting the, 3–4
        defining the purpose of, 2
        in delirium, 12–16
        in dementia, 4–8
        in depression, 8–12
        interpreting the results of, 4
        selecting the instrument for, 2–3

D

Delirium, in older persons, 12–16
        clinical features, 13–15
        cognitive assessment, 15–16
        epidemiology, 12–13
        risk factors, 15
Dementia, 1–129
    Alzheimer's disease, abuse and neglect
        of older adults with, **43–55**
            assessment of, 47–50
            barriers to detection and
                intervention, 51
            elder mistreatment, 43–44
            prevention and treatment
                of, 50–51
            reciprocal violence, 46–47
            risk factors for, 44–46
            vulnerability in, 44
    measuring quality of nursing care
        for patients with, **95–104**
    practical orientation to,
        119–127
            checklists for early detection
                of, 123, 124
            criteria for diagnosis of, 125
            dementia as a class of brain
                disease, 120–121
            key functions disrupted by
                dementia in, 122
            model for progression of, 126
    primary care and, issues and
        challenges in, **83–95**
            clinical dilemmas, 83
            family caregivers, 87, 91
            pharmacologic interventions,
                91
            screening, 84–87
            stage-based nursing
                interventions for, 92–93
            staging, 87, 88–90
    clinical features, 5–6
    cognitive assessment, **1–22**
        conducting the, 3–4
        defining the purpose of, 2
        in delirium, 12–16
        in dementia, 4–8
        in depression, 8–12
        interpreting the results of, 4
        selecting the instrument for, 2–3

    drug therapy for, research methods to
        study efficacy-effectiveness gap in,
        105–117
        background, 107–109
        example of, 109–115
        nurses' role in, 115–116
    epidemiology, 4–5
    progressively lowered stress threshold
        model in, **57–81**
        application of, across continuum of
            care, 61–79
        overview, 57–61
    psychoemotional and behavioral status
        in patients with, **23–41**
        assessment of depression in
            nursing homes, 31–32
        behavioral assessment, 32–36
        depression in older adults, key
            components of, 23–27
            anxiety, 26
            appetite impairment, 26
            disagreeable behavior,
                25–26
            lack of meaning in life, 26–27
            melancholic behavior, 25
            sleep impairment, 26
        individualized care for older adults
            with dementia who are
            depressed, 32
        instrumentation in assessment of,
            27–31
        issues related to, 36–38
    risk factors, 6
Depression, in older persons, 8–12
        clinical features, 8–10
        cognitive assessment, 11–12
        epidemiology, 8
        risk factors, 10–11
    psychoemotional and behavioral status
        of older patients with dementia,
        23–41
        assessment of, in nursing homes,
            31–32
        behavioral assessment, 32–36
        individualized care for older adults
            with dementia who are
            depressed, 32
        instrumentation in assessment of,
            27–31
        issues related to, 36–38
        key components of, 23–27
            anxiety, 26
            appetite impairment, 26
            disagreeable behavior, 25–26
            lack of meaning in life, 26–27
            melancholic behavior, 25
            sleep impairment, 26
Disagreeable behavior, in older adults with
    dementia, 25–26

Drug therapy, for Alzheimer's patients, 91
    research methods to study efficacy-
        effectiveness gap in, **105–117**
        background, 105–109
        example of, for mild to moderate
            dementia, 109–115
        nurses' role in, 115–116

E

Eden Alternative nursing facility,
    progressively lowered stress threshold
    care plan for dementia in, 76–77
Efficacy-effectiveness gap, in drug therapy for
    dementia, longitudinal observational
    studies of, **105–117**
Elder mistreatment, abuse and neglect of
    older adults with Alzheimer's disease,
    43–55
        assessment of, 47–50
        barriers to detection and
            intervention, 51
        prevention and treatment of,
            50–51
        reciprocal violence, 46–47
        risk factors for, 44–46
        vulnerability in, 44

F

Family caregivers, of Alzheimer's patients, 87,
    91
        stage-based nursing interventions
            for, 92–93
FExT Study, 111–117

H

Home care, progressively lowered stress
    threshold care plan for dementia in,
    64–66
Hopelessness, lack of meaning in life of older
    adults with dementia, 26–27
Hospitalization, progressively lowered stress
    threshold care plan for dementia care
    during, 73–75

L

Longitudinal observational studies, of
    efficacy-effectiveness gap in drug
    therapy for mild and moderate
    dementia, **105–117**
        background, 107–109
        example of, 109–115
        nurses' role in, 115–116

M

Measurement, of quality of nursing care to
    Alzheimer's patients, **95–104**

Melancholic behavior, in older adults with
    dementia, 25

N

Neglect, of older persons. *See* Elder
    mistreatment.
Nursing care, for Alzheimer's patients,
    measuring quality of, **95–104**

O

Observational studies, longitudinal, of
    efficacy-effectiveness gap in drug
    therapy for mild and moderate
    dementia, **105–117**
Older adults, dementia and depression in.
    See Dementia *and* Depression.
Outcomes, measuring quality of nursing care
    to patients with, **95–104**

P

Pharmacologic interventions. *See* Drug
    therapy.
Primary care, Alzheimer's disease and, issues
    and challenges in, **83–93**
        clinical dilemmas, 83
        family caregivers, 87, 91
        pharmacologic interventions, 91
        screening, 84–87
        stage-based nursing interventions
            for, 92–93
        staging, 87, 88–90
Progressively lowered stress threshold model,
    57–81
        application of, across continuum of
            dementia care, 61–79
            for assisted living care, 68–70
            for Eden Alternative nursing
                facility, 76–77
            for home care, 64–66
            for hospital care, 73–75
        for dementia, overview of, 57–61
Psychoemotional status, and behavioral status
    in older patients with dementia,
    23–41
        assessment of depression in
            nursing homes, 31–32
        behavioral assessment, 32–36
        depression in older adults, key
            components of, 23–27
            anxiety, 26
            appetite impairment, 26
            disagreeable behavior, 25–26
            lack of meaning in life, 26–27
            melancholic behavior, 25
            sleep impairment, 26

Psychoemotional (*continued*)
> individualized care for older adults with dementia who are depressed, 32
> instrumentation in assessment of, 27–31
> issues related to, 36–38

Q

Quality, of nursing care, for Alzheimer's patients, measurement of, **95–104**

R

Reciprocal violence, committed by caregivers of Alzheimer's patients, 46–47

Research methods, longitudinal observational studies of efficacy-effectiveness gap in drug therapy for dementia, **105–117**
measuring quality of nursing care to Alzheimer's patients, **95–104**

Rivastigmine, study of efficacy-effectiveness gap in mild to moderate dementia, 109–115

S

Screening, in primary care practice, for Alzheimer's disease, 84–87
> brief cognitive tests, 85
> functional and behavioral assessment, 85–87

Sleep impairment, in older adults with dementia, 26

Staging, of Alzheimer's disease, 87, 88–90

Stress, application of progressively lowered stress threshold model in dementia care, **57–81**

V

Violence, reciprocal, committed by caregivers of Alzheimer's patients, 46–47

Changing Your Address?

Make sure your subscription changes too! When you notify us of your new address, you can help make our job easier by including an exact copy of your Clinics label number with your old address (see illustration below.) This number identifies you to our computer system and will speed the processing of your address change. Please be sure this label number accompanies your old address and your corrected address—you can send an old Clinics label with your number on it or just copy it exactly and send it to the address listed below.

We appreciate your help in our attempt to give you continuous coverage. Thank you.

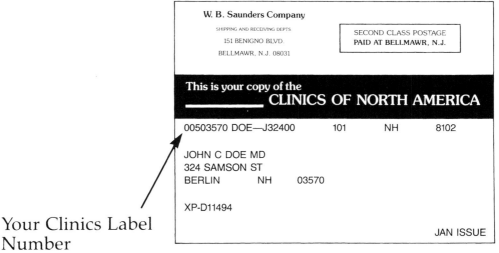

Your Clinics Label Number

Copy it exactly or send your label along with your address to:
W.B. Saunders Company, Customer Service
Orlando, FL 32887-4800
Call Toll Free 1-800-654-2452

Please allow four to six weeks for delivery of new subscriptions and for processing address changes.